medical abbreviations handbook

second edition

Originally published as
Quick Directory of Medical Abbreviations

MEDICAL ECONOMICS BOOKS
Oradell, New Jersey 07649

Library of Congress Cataloging in Publication Data

Main entry under title:

Medical abbreviations handbook.

   1. Medicine—Abbreviations.   I. Patient care.
(DNLM: 1. Abbreviations—Dictionaries.   2. Medicine—
Abbreviations.   W 13 Q6)
R123.M387 1983   610'.148   82-20399
ISBN 0-87489-309-7

ISBN 0-87489-309-7

Medical Economics Company Inc.
Oradell, New Jersey 07649

Printed in the United States of America

contents

1/85

acknowledgments

This book has been adapted and expanded from compilations supplied by the medical record departments of the following:

University Hospital, University of Colorado, Denver

Hahnemann University Hospital, Philadelphia

Henry Ford Hospital, Detroit

University Hospital, University of Washington, Seattle

Yale-New Haven Hospital, New Haven, Conn.

introduction

Medical Abbreviations Handbook began as a series in *Patient Care* magazine—eight installments covering nine subject areas: anatomic terms, physiologic terms, symptoms and diseases, diagnostic terms, therapeutic terms, orders/instructions, medical chemistry, terms of measurement, and organisms.

As with many articles in *Patient Care*, this idea was generated by a reader. Several years ago, *Patient Care* sent a draft of an article on disseminated intravascular coagulation to a number of physicians for prepublication review. The abbreviation "DIC" appeared throughout the article, spurring one reviewer to comment that he would find a list of such abbreviations very useful. Additional research found that most *Patient Care* readers agreed. So the staff at *Patient Care* set to work compiling such a list—the first of a series to include nearly all categories of abbreviations used in medicine.

Medical record departments of several hospitals were asked to supply lists of abbreviations they used regularly. The lists were used in developing the series.

The first installment was published in May, 1975; the eighth in July, 1976. Ever since the first list appeared, the publishers have had a hard time keeping up with requests for reprints from physicians, nurses, physician's assistants, directors of hospital medical record departments, clinic managers, and others involved directly and indirectly with medical records. For this reason, the series was published in book form.

The first book edition, entitled *Quick Directory of Medical Abbreviations,* proved to be as popular as the series: Two printings were sold out. This new book has been updated, revised, and expanded by Logical Communications Inc. (formerly the book division of Patient Care), with the cooperation of the medical record librarians at the hospitals listed in the Acknowledgments. Nearly 10 percent more abbreviations have been added.

anatomic terms

A, α	anterior artery axial
AA	alveolar-arterial arteries ascending aorta
AAL	anterior axillary line
ABD, abd	abdomen
AC	acromioclavicular adrenal cortex atriocarotid auriculocarotid
AD, ad	right ear *(auris dextra)*
ADA	anterior descending artery
AE	above the elbow
AF	amniotic fluid aortic flow
AFP	anterior faucial pillar
AK, ak	above knee
ALH	anterior lobe of the hypophysis
ALN	anterior lymph node
ALW	arch-loop-whorl
AN	anterior

ANS	autonomic nervous system
ANT, ant	anterior
AO, Ao	aorta
AP	anterior pituitary
	appendix
AP, A-P	anteroposterior
A&P	anterior and posterior
APC	adenoidal-pharyngeal-conjunctival
APP	appendix
ART, art	artery
AS, as	left ear *(auris sinistra)*
ASIS	anterior superior iliac spine
ASS	anterior superior spine
AU	both ears *(aures unitas)*
aur	ear *(auris)*
AV, A-V	arteriovenous
	atrioventricular
	atrioventricular node
AVN	atrioventricular node
AW	anterior wall
Ax	axilla
	axillary
B	buccal
BA	brachial artery
BB	both bones
BBB	blood-brain barrier
BC	Bowman's capsule
BD	bile duct

BE	below the elbow
BH	bundle of His
BIL, Bil	bilateral
BJM	bones, joints, and muscles
BK	below knee
BLN	bronchial lymph nodes
BM	basement membrane bone marrow
BMK	birthmark
BP	bronchopleural
BUS	Bartholin's, urethral, and Skene's glands
BV	blood vessel bronchovesicular
C	cervical chest
C$_1$, C$_2$	first cervical vertebra, second, etc.
C$_I$, C$_{II}$	first cranial nerve, second, etc.
CA	coronary artery
CBD	common bile duct
CC	coracoclavicular corpus callosum costochondral
CCA	common carotid artery
CD	common duct conjugata diagonalis cystic duct
CD, cd	caudal
CDS	cul-de-sac

CF	chest and left leg
ch	chest
cl	corpus luteum
CL	chest and left arm
CM	costal margin
CN	cranial nerves
CNS	central nervous system
COC, Coc	coccygeal
COR, cor	heart
CR	cardiorespiratory
	chest and right arm
Cr$_1$, Cr$_2$	first cranial nerve, second, etc.
CRA	central retinal artery
cr ns	cranial nerves
CRV	central retinal vein
CS	coronary sinus
	corpus striatum
CSF	cerebrospinal fluid
CSN	carotid sinus nerve
CT	connective tissue
CV	cardiovascular
	central venous
	cerebrovascular
CVA, cva	costovertebral angle
CVR	cardiovascular-renal
	cardiovascular-respiratory
CVS	cardiovascular system
CW	chest wall
CX, Cx	cervix

D	dorsal
D, d	distal
D_1, D_2	first dorsal vertebra, second, etc.
DA	ductus arteriosus
DIP	distal interphalangeal
DIPJ	distal interphalangeal joint
DP	dorsalis pedis
E	eye
EAC	external auditory canal
EAM	external auditory meatus
EC	extracellular
ECF	extracellular fluid
ECM	extracellular material
ECW	extracellular water
EE	eye and ear
EENT	eye, ear, nose, and throat
EHC	enterohepatic circulation
EIP	extensor indicis proprius
ENT	ear, nose, and throat
EOM	extraocular muscles or motion
ESO	esophagus
ET	endotracheal eustachian tube
EV	extravascular
EXT, ext	external
extr	extremity
F	finger foramen

FA	femoral artery
	forearm
fem	femoral or femur
FH	fetal head
	fetal heart
FHT	fetal heart
FO	foramen ovale
	fronto-occipital
FP	frontoparietal
F-P	femoral popliteal
G	gingival
GALT	gut-associated lymphoid tissue
GB	gallbladder
GBM	glomerular basement membrane
GC	ganglion cells
GI	gastrointestinal
GIS	gastrointestinal system
GIT	gastrointestinal tract
GL	gland
GM	gastric mucosa
GU	genitourinary
GUS	genitourinary system
HA	hepatic artery
hd	head
HEENT	head, eyes, ears, nose, and throat
H&L	heart and lungs
HLK	heart, liver, kidney
HN	hilar node

HT, Ht	heart
HV	hepatic vein
I	permanent incisor
IA	internal auditory intra-aortic intra-arterial
IAC	internal auditory canal
IAM	internal auditory meatus
IAS	interatrial septum
IC	intercostal internal capsule intracellular intracerebral intracarotid intracranial intracutaneous
ICF	intracellular fluid
ICM	intercostal margin
ICS	intercostal space
ICW	intracellular water
ID	intraduodenal
ID, id	intradermal
IF	interstitial fluid
IG	intragastric
IM	intramedullary intramuscular
IMA	internal mammary artery
IN	intranasal
Ing	inguinal

IO	internal os intraocular
IP	interphalangeal intraperitoneal
IPL	intrapleural
IS	intercostal space
ISF	interstitial fluid
ISW	interstitial water
IT	intratracheal
IU	intrauterine
IV	intravascular intravenous intraventricular intravertebral
IVag	intravaginal
IVC	inferior vena cava
IVD	intervertebral disk
IVS	interventricular septum
JEJ, Jej	jejunum
JG	juxtaglomerular
JGC	juxtaglomerular cell
JT, jt	joint
JV	jugular vein
JVP	jugular vein pulse
K	calix kidney
KLS	kidney, liver, spleen
KN	knee
KUB	kidney, ureter, and bladder

KUS	kidney, ureter, and spleen
L	ligament
	liver
	lumbar
LA	left arm
	left atrium
	left auricle
LCA	left coronary artery
LCM	left costal margin
LD	left deltoid
LE	left eye
	lower extremity
LES	lower esophageal sphincter
LFA	left femoral artery
LG	left gluteal
LHL	left hepatic lobe
LICS	left intercostal space
LIF	left iliac fossa
Lig	ligament
LIQ	lower inner quadrant
LIR	left iliac region
LIS	left intercostal space
LIV	left innominate vein
LK	left kidney
LKS	liver, kidneys, and spleen
LL	left leg
	left lower
	left lung
	lower lobe

LLE	left lower extremity
LLL	left lower leg
	left lower lobe
	left lower lung
LLQ	left lower quadrant
LLR	left lumbar region
LMCA	left middle cerebral artery
LN	lymph node
LOQ	lower outer quadrant
LPA	left pulmonary artery
LPV	left pulmonary veins
LRQ	lower right quadrant
LRT	lower respiratory tract
LS	left side
	liver and spleen
	lumbosacral
LSB	left sternal border
LSK	liver, spleen, and kidneys
L-sp	lumbar spine
LSV	left subclavian vein
LT	left thigh
LU	left upper
LUE	left upper extremity
LUL	left upper lobe
	left upper lung
lumb	lumbar
LUQ	left upper quadrant
LV	left ventricle

L_1, L_2	first lumbar vertebra or nerve, second, etc.
M, m	muscle
MAL	midaxillary line
MC	metacarpal
MCA	middle cerebral artery
MCL	midclavicular line midcostal line
MCP	metacarpophalangeal
ME	middle ear
MG	muscle group
ML	middle lobe midline
MM	medial malleolus mucous membrane muscles muscularis mucosae
MN	motor neuron myoneural
MP	metacarpophalangeal metaphalangeal metatarsophalangeal
MPA	main pulmonary artery
MPJ	metacarpophalangeal joint
MS	musculoskeletal
MSL	midsternal line
MT	membrana tympani metatarsal muscles and tendons
MTP	metatarsophalangeal

MV	mitral valve
N	nasal
	nerve
NE	nerve ending
NG, ng	nasogastric
NM	neuromuscular
NMJ	neuromuscular junction
NP	nasopharynx
Ns	nerves
NS	nervous system
NT	nasotracheal
N + T	nose and throat
O	eye
O₂	both eyes
occ	occiput, occipital
OD, od	right eye *(oculus dexter)*
OFC	occipitofrontal circumference
OFD	oral-facial-digital
OL	left eye *(oculus laevus)*
OS, os	left eye *(oculus sinister)*
	mouth
OT	orotracheal
OU, ou	both eyes *(oculi unitas)*
OURQ	outer upper right quadrant
Ov	ovary
P	pupil
PA	pulmonary artery
PAL	posterior axillary line

PC	portacaval
	pulmonary capillary
PCA	posterior cerebral artery
PCF	posterior cranial fossa
PE	pharyngoesophageal
per	perineal
PIP	proximal interphalangeal
PIPJ	proximal interphalangeal joint
pl	platelets
	pleural
PLV	posterior left ventricle
PN	peripheral nerve
PNS	peripheral nervous system
PP	proximal phalanx
PSL	parasternal line
PT	parathyroid
	posterior tibial
PUL, PULM	pulmonary
PV	peripheral vein
	portal vein
R, (R)	rectal
RA	renal artery
	right arm
	right atrial
	right atrium
	right auricle
RBC	red blood cell
	red blood corpuscle
RC	red cell
RCA	right coronary artery

RCM	right costal margin
RD	right deltoid
RE	reticuloendothelial
	right eye
REG UMB	umbilical region
REN	renal
RES	reticuloendothelial system
RFA	right femoral artery
RG	right gluteal
RHL	right hepatic lobe
RHLN	right hilar lymph node
RIF	right iliac fossa
RIR	right iliac region
RL	right leg
	right lung
RLE	right lower extremity
RLL	right lower lobe
RLN	recurrent laryngeal nerve
RLQ	right lower quadrant
RMCA	right middle cerebral artery
RML	right middle lobe
RML, rml	right mediolateral
ROP	right occipitoposterior
ROT	right occipitotransverse
RPA	right pulmonary artery
RPV	right pulmonary veins
RSV	right subclavian vein
RT	right thigh

RUE	right upper extremity
RUL	right upper lobe
	right upper lung
RUQ	right upper quadrant
RV	right ventricle
S	sacral
S_1, S_2	first sacral vertebra or nerve, second, etc.
SA, S-A	sinoatrial
SB	small bowel
	sternal border
SC	sacrococcygeal
	sternoclavicular
	subcutaneous
SCM	sternocleidomastoid
SF	spinal fluid
SH	shoulder
SI	sacroiliac
SIJ	sacroiliac joint
SLN	superior laryngeal nerve
SMA	superior mesenteric artery
SN	suprasternal notch
SNS	sympathetic nervous system
SP	spine
	suprapubic
	symphysis pubis
sp cd	spinal cord
sp fl	spinal fluid
SQ, sq	subcutaneous

st	stomach
ST	sternothyroid
sub-q	subcutaneous
SV	subclavian vein
SVC	superior vena cava
T	thoracic
T_1, T_2; T1, T2	first thoracic (dorsal) vertebra or nerve, second, etc.
T&A	tonsils and adenoids
TBM	tubular basement membrane
TD	thoracic duct
TDL	thoracic duct lymph
TE	tracheoesophageal
TH	thyrohyoid
TH, th	thoracic
TIVC	thoracic inferior vena cava
TM	temporomandibular transmetatarsal tympanic membrane
TMJ	temporomandibular joint
TO	tubo-ovarian
TP	posterior tibial
TT	transthoracic
UA	umbilical artery
UB	ultimobranchial body
UE	upper extremity
UES	upper esophageal sphincter
UG	urogenital

UGI	upper gastrointestinal
UIQ	upper inner quadrant
UL	upper lobe
ULQ	upper left quadrant
UO	ureteral orifice
UOQ	upper outer quadrant
UP	ureteropelvic
UPJ	ureteropelvic junction
UR	upper respiratory
UR, ur	urine
URQ	upper right quadrant
UV	umbilical vein
UVJ	ureterovesical junction
V	vein
VA	ventriculoatrial vertebral artery
VAG, Vag	vagina, vaginal
VASC	vascular
VC	vena cava vocal cord
VENT	ventricular
vent	ventral
VES	bladder *(vesica)* vesicular
VM	ventricular muscle
VV, vv	veins
VW	vessel wall
WB	whole blood whole body

WBC white blood cell
       white blood corpuscle
WC white cell
WR wrist

physiologic terms

A_2	second aortic sound
$A_2 > P_2$	second aortic greater than second pulmonic
$A_2 < P_2$	second aortic less than second pulmonic
A-a	alveolar-arterial (gradient)
A-ao$_2$	alveolar-arterial O_2 (gradient)
A/B	acid-base ratio
ABP	arterial blood pressure
AC	anodal closure aortic closure
A/C	albumin-coagulin ratio
ACC	anodal closing contraction
ACCL	anodal closure clonus
ACD	anterior chest diameter
ACO	anodal closing odor
ACP	anodal closing picture
ACS	anodal closing sound
ACTe	anodal closure tetanus
AD	anodal duration
ADC	anodal duration contraction
ADP	area diastolic pressure

A-DV	arterio-deep venous difference
AER	aldosterone excretion rate
AF	aortic flow
A/G, A-G, A/G Ratio	albumin-globulin ratio
AIP	average intravascular pressure
AJ	ankle jerk
ALB/GLOB	albumin-globulin ratio
AMP	average mean pressure
ANCC	anodal closing contraction
Ang GR	angiotensin generation rate
ANOC	anodal opening contraction
AO	anodal opening aortic opening opening of the atrioventricular valves
AOC	anodal opening contraction
AOCL	anodal opening clonus
AOO	anodal opening odor
AOP	anodal opening picture
AoP	left ventricle to aorta pressure gradient
AOS	anodal opening sound
AOTe	anodal opening tetanus
AP	apical pulse arterial pressure
A/P	ascites-plasma ratio
APGL	alkaline phosphatase activity of the granular leukocytes

ASP	area systolic pressure
ASR	aldosterone secretion rate
A-SV	arterio-superficial venous difference
ATR	Achilles tendon reflex
A-Vo$_2$	arteriovenous oxygen difference
A/V ratio	ratio of the size of arterioles to venules
BA	bacterial agglutination brachial arterial (pressure)
BAC	blood alcohol concentration
BAm	mean brachial artery (pressure)
BAO	basal acid output
BASH	body acceleration given synchronously with the heartbeat
BBT	basal body temperature
BC	bone conduction (ear)
BF	blood flow
B/F	bound-free ratio
BFR	blood flow rate bone formation rate
BH/VH	body hematocrit-venous hematocrit ratio
bisp	bispinous or interspinous diameter
BJ	biceps jerk
BL PR	blood pressure
BM	bowel movement

BMR	basal metabolic rate
BP	blood pressure
BPD	blood pressure decreased
BPI	blood pressure increased
BRP	bilirubin production
BS, bs	breath sounds
BSA	body surface area
BTR	Bezold-type reflex
BV	blood volume
BW	birth weight body water body weight
C	clearance rate
CACC	cathodal closing contraction
CADTe	cathodal duration tetanus
CBF	capillary blood flow cerebral blood flow coronary blood flow
CBV	central blood volume circulating blood volume corrected blood volume
CC	circulatory collapse
CCC	cathodal closing contraction
CCCL	cathodal closure clonus
CCTe	cathodal closure tetanus
CD	conjugata diagonalis
CF	coronary flow
CG/OQ	cerebral glucose oxygen quotient
CH	crown-heel (length of fetus)

CIRC, Circ	circulation
CMO	cardiac minute output
CMR	cerebral metabolic rate
CMRG	cerebral metabolic rate of glucose
CMRO	cerebral metabolic rate of oxygen
CO	cardiac output
COAG	coagulation
COC, COCL	cathodal opening clonus
CP	capillary pressure
C/P	cholesterol-phospholipid ratio
CPAP	continuous positive airway pressure
CPPB	continuous positive pressure breathing
CPR	cerebral cortex perfusion rate cortisol production rate
CR	conditioned reflex crown-rump (length of fetus)
CSR	cortisol secretion rate
CT	cardiothoracic
CTR	cardiothoracic ratio
CV	cell volume conjugate diameter of pelvic inlet *(conjugata vera)* corpuscular volume
CVA	costovertebral angle

CVO	obstetric conjugate diameter of pelvic inlet *(conjugata vera obstetrica)*
CVP	central venous pressure
CVR	cerebral vascular resistance
D_1	inulin dialysance
D_{CO}	diffusing capacity for carbon monoxide
D_L	diffusing capacity of the lung
D_U	urea dialysance
DA	direct agglutination
DBP	diastolic blood pressure
def	defecation
DF	dorsiflexion
DL	diffusing capacity of the lung
DLCO	diffusing capacity of the lung for carbon monoxide
D/N	dextrose-nitrogen ratio
DOC-SR	desoxycorticosterone secretion rate
DP	diastolic pressure
DS	duration of systole
DSVP	downstream venous pressure
DTR	deep tendon reflex
EC	excitation-contraction
ECBV	effective circulating blood volume
ECF	effective capillary flow
ECFV	extracellular fluid volume

ECV	extracellular volume
	extracorporeal volume
ECVE	extracellular volume expansion
EDP	end-diastolic pressure
EDV	end-diastolic volume
EEEP	end-expiratory esophageal pressure
EFR	effective filtration rate
EFV	extracellular fluid volume
EFVC	expiratory flow-volume curve
EHBF	estimated hepatic blood flow
	exercise hyperemia blood flow
EHC	enterohepatic circulation
E/I	expiration-inspiration ratio
EJ	elbow jerk
ERBF	effective renal blood flow
ERPF	effective renal plasma flow
ERV	expiratory reserve volume
ESP	end-systolic pressure
ESR	erythrocyte sedimentation rate
ESV	end-systolic volume
ETP	eustachian tube pressure
EXBF	exercise hyperemia blood flow
expir	expiration
FBF	forearm blood flow
FBP	femoral blood pressure
FECV	functional extracellular fluid volume
FEF	forced expiratory flow
FEV	forced expiratory volume

FEV$_1$	forced expiratory volume in one second
FEV$_1$/VC	forced expiratory volume (in one second)/vital capacity
FHR	fetal heart rate
FHS	fetal heart sounds
FHT	fetal heart tones
FHVP	free hepatic vein pressure
Fib	fibrillation
FIF	forced inspiratory flow
FIFR	fasting intestinal flow rate
FIO$_2$	fractional inspired oxygen
flex	flexion
FRC	functional reserve capacity functional residual capacity
FVC	forced vital capacity
FVE	forced expiratory volume
FVR	forearm vascular resistances
G/E	granulocyte-erythroid ratio
GET	gastric emptying time
GET$^{1/2}$	gastric emptying half-time
GFR	glomerular filtration rate
G/N	glucose-nitrogen ratio
HA	hemagglutination
HABF	hepatic artery blood flow
HBF	hand blood flow hepatic blood flow
HC	head circumference heart cycle

HD	hearing distance
HM	hand movement(s)
HMO	heart minute output
HMP	hexose monophosphate pathway
HR, HRT	heart rate
IBC	iron-binding capacity
IC	inspiratory capacity
ICT	isovolumic contraction time
IDP	instantaneous diastolic pressure
I/E	inspiratory-expiratory ratio
IFR	inspiratory flow rate
IFV	intracellular fluid volume
IGV	intrathoracic gas volume
IHA	indirect hemagglutination
IHR	intrahepatic resistance intrinsic heart rate
IJP	internal jugular pressure
IMBC	indirect maximum breathing capacity
IO	incisal opening
IOP	intraocular pressure
IPP	intrapleural pressure
IPSP	inhibitory postsynaptic potential
IRV	inspiratory reserve volume
ISA$_5$	internal surface area of lung at volume of 5 liters
IVC	isovolumic contraction period
IVCP	inferior vena cava pressure

IVPF	isovolumic pressure flow
IVR	isovolumic relaxation time
JGI	juxtaglomerular granulation index
	juxtaglomerular index
JJ	jaw jerk
JVP	jugular venous pulse
KC	kathodal (cathodal) closing
KCC	kathodal (cathodal) closing contraction
KD	kathodal (cathodal) duration
KJ	knee jerk
KK	knee kick
KOC	kathodal (cathodal) opening contraction
KSC	kathodal (cathodal) closing contraction
LAP	left atrial pressure
lact	lactating
LBNP	lower-body negative pressure
LBW	low birth weight
LBWR	lung-body weight ratio
LIBC	latent iron-binding capacity
LLM	localized leukocyte mobilization
LMP	last menstrual period
LNMP	last normal menstrual period
LP	light perception
L/P	liver to plasma concentration ratio
	lymph-plasma ratio
LPR	lactate-pyruvate ratio

L/S ratio	lecithin/sphingomyelin ratio
LV	lung volume
LV_D	left ventricular end-diastolic pressure
LVDP	left ventricular diastolic pressure
LVDV	left ventricular diastolic volume
LVEDC	left ventricular end-diastolic circumference
LVEDP	left ventricular end-diastolic pressure
LVEDV	left ventricular end-diastolic volume
LVEP	left ventricular end-diastolic pressure
LVET	left ventricular ejection time
LVP	left ventricular pressure
LVs	mean left ventricular systolic pressure
LVSP	left ventricular systolic pressure
LVSV	left ventricular stroke volume
LVSW	left ventricular stroke work
LVT	left ventricular tension
LVW	left ventricular work
LVWI	left ventricular work index
M-1	first mitral sound
ma	meter-angle
MA	mean arterial (blood pressure) muscle activity
MABP	mean arterial blood pressure

MAC	minimum alveolar concentration
MAP	mean aortic pressure mean arterial pressure muscle-action potential
Max EP	maximum esophageal pressure
MBC	maximum breathing capacity
MBF	myocardial blood flow
MBP	mean blood pressure
MCBR	minimum concentration of bilirubin
MCC	mean corpuscular hemoglobin concentration
MCD	mean cell diameter mean corpuscular diameter
MCF	myocardial contractile force
MCHC	mean corpuscular hemoglobin concentration
MCI	mean cardiac index
MCR	metabolic clearance rate
MCS	myocardial contractile state
MCT	mean circulation time mean corpuscular thickness
MCV	mean cell volume mean corpuscular volume
MDA	motor discriminative acuity
M/E	myeloid-erythroid ratio
MEF	maximum expiratory flow
MEFR	maximum expiratory flow rate
MEFSR	maximum expiratory flow— static recoil curve

MEFV	maximum expiratory flow volume
MFR	mucus flow rate
MGP	marginal granulocyte pool
MHR	maximal heart rate
MIFR	maximum inspiratory flow rate
MIP	maximum inspiratory pressure
	mean intravascular pressure
M:L	monocyte-lymphocyte ratio
MLAP	mean left atrial pressure
MMEF, MMEFR	maximum midexpiratory flow rate
MMF	maximum midexpiratory flow
MMFR	maximum midexpiratory flow rate
	maximum midflow rate
MMR	myocardial metabolic rate
MNCV	motor nerve conduction velocity
MO_2	myocardial oxygen consumption
MP	menstrual period
MPAP	mean pulmonary arterial pressure
MR	metabolic rate
MRAP	mean right atrial pressure

MRF	mitral regurgitant flow
MRVP	mean right ventricular pressure
MSER	mean systolic ejection rate
MVC	myocardial vascular capacity
MV grad	mitral valve gradient
MVO_2	myocardial oxygen consumption
MVV	maximum voluntary ventilation
MVV_1	maximal ventilatory volume
NLP	normal light perception
NMP	normal menstrual period
NON-REM	nonrapid eye movement
NRC	normal retinal correspondence
NREM	nonrapid eye movement
NSR	normal sinus rhythm
NTP	normal temperature and pressure
NVA	near visual acuity
O_2 CAP	oxygen capacity
OFC	occipitofrontal circumference
OP	osmotic pressure
P	pulse
P_{BA}	brachial arterial pressure
P_L	pulmonary venous pressure
P_{Pa}	pulmonary artery pressure
P_2, P-2	pulmonic second sound
P_{TP}	transpulmonary pressure

Pa_{CO_2}	arterial carbon dioxide pressure, tension
PA_{CO_2}	alveolar CO_2 pressure, tension
PACP	pulmonary artery counter-pulsation
PA_{O_2}	alveolar O_2 pressure, tension
Pa_{O_2}	arterial oxygen pressure
PAP	pulmonary artery pressure
PAR	pulmonary arteriolar resistance
PBF	pulmonary blood flow
PBV	predicted blood volume pulmonary blood volume
PC	pulmonic closure
Pco	carbon monoxide pressure, tension
PCO_2, pCO_2	carbon dioxide pressure
PCV	packed cell volume
PD	papilla diameter pupillary distance
p.d.	papilla diameter
PEF	peak expiratory flow
PEFR	peak expiratory flow rate
PEFSR	partial expiratory flow—static recoil curve
PEFV	partial expiratory flow volume
PGDR	plasma glucose disappearance rate
PGTR	plasma glucose tolerance rate

PIA	plasma insulin activity
PIDT	plasma iron disappearance time
PIF	peak inspiratory flow
PIFR	peak inspiratory flow rate
PIT	plasma iron turnover
PITR	plasma iron turnover rate
PK	psychokinesis
PL	perception of light
PMI	point of maximal impulse point of maximum impulse
PMP	past menstrual period previous menstrual period
PMTT	pulmonary mean transit time
PNS	peripheral nerve stimulator
PO_2	arterial oxygen pressure
po_2	partial pressure of oxygen
POP	plasma oncotic pressure
PP	pulse pressure
post. sag. D	posterior sagittal diameter
PPBS	postprandial blood sugar
PR	pulse rate
PRA	plasma renin activity
PRBV	placental residual blood volume
PRHBF	peak reactive hyperemia blood flow
PSG	peak systolic gradient
psp	postsynaptic potential

PSR	extrahepatic portal-systemic resistance
PTHS	parathyroid hormone secretion (rate)
PV	plasma volume
Pvco_2	venous carbon dioxide pressure
PVF	portal venous flow
PVP	portal venous pressure
PVR	peripheral vascular resistance pulmonary vascular resistance
PWC	physical work capacity
Qc	pulmonary capillary blood flow
Qo_2	oxygen consumption
R	respiration
R_A	airway resistance
R_L, R_P	pulmonary resistance
R_T	total pulmonary resistance
RAD	right axis deviation
RAIU	radioactive iodine uptake
RAM	rapid alternating movements
RAP	right atrial pressure
RBCV	red blood cell volume
RBF	renal blood flow
RCBV	regional cerebral blood volume
RCD	relative cardiac dullness
RCV	red cell volume
RD	reaction of degeneration
RDI	rupture-delivery interval

REM	rapid eye movement
RER	renal excretion rate
RESP, Resp	respiration
RF	relative flow rate
RHBF	reactive hyperemia blood flow
RHD	relative hepatic dullness
RLC	residual lung capacity
RM	respiratory movement
RMD	right manubrial dullness
RMV	respiratory minute volume
ROM	range of motion
RPF	renal plasma flow
RR	respiratory rate
RRR	renin-release rate
RSR	regular sinus rhythm
RV	residual volume respiratory volume
RVDV	right ventricular diastolic volume
RVEDP	right ventricular end-diastolic pressure
RVR	renal vascular resistance resistance to venous return
RVRA	renal vein renin activity
RVRC	renal vein renin concentration
RV/TLC	residual volume-total lung capacity ratio
S_1, S_2	first, second heart sounds

S_3	third heart sound ventricular gallop sound
Sao_2	oxygen percent saturation (arterial)
SAP	systemic arterial pressure
SBF	splanchnic blood flow
SBP	systemic blood pressure systolic blood pressure
SC	closure of the semilunar valves
S/D	systolic to diastolic
SDA	specific dynamic action
SEP	systolic ejection period
SER	systolic ejection rate
SET	systolic ejection time
SFP	spinal fluid pressure
SFT	skinfold thickness
SGFR	single-nephron glomerular filtration rate
SHHP	semihorizontal heart position
SMR	somnolent metabolic rate
SP	systolic pressure
SR	sinus rhythm stretch reflex
ST	sphincter tone
SV	stroke volume
SVI	stroke volume index
SVR	systemic vascular resistance
SW	stroke work
SWI	stroke work index

T	tension, intraocular
TBD	total body density
TBF	total body fat
TBI	thyrobinding index
TBK	total body potassium
TBV	total blood volume
TBVp	total blood volume predicted from body surface
TBW	total body water total body weight
TCF	total coronary flow
TCH	total circulating hemoglobin
TCNS	transcutaneous nerve stimulator
TDF	thoracic duct flow
TDP	thoracic duct pressure
TENS	transelectrical nerve stimulator
TF	tactile fremitus
TGV	thoracic gas volume
TIBC	total iron-binding capacity
TJ	triceps jerk
TLC	total lung capacity
Tm	maximal tubular excretory capacity of the kidneys
TmG	maximal tubular reabsorption rate of glucose
Tn	normal intraocular tension
TNR	tonic neck reflex
TPBF	total pulmonary blood flow

TPR	temperature, pulse, respiration testosterone production rate total peripheral resistance total pulmonary resistance
TPTHS	total parathyroid hormone secretion rate
TPVR	total pulmonary vascular resistance
TR	tubular reabsorption
TRBF	total renal blood flow
TRP	tubular reabsorption of phosphate
TSP	total serum protein
TSPAP	total serum prostatic acid phosphatase
TSR	thyroid-serum ratio
TV	tidal volume
TVC	timed vital capacity total volume capacity
UA/C	uric acid-creatinine ratio
UBBC	unsaturated vitamin B_{12}-binding capacity
UBF	uterine blood flow
UBP	ureteral back pressure
UIBC	unsaturated iron-binding capacity
Umax	maximum urinary osmolality
Uosm	urinary osmolality
U/P	urine-plasma ratio
UV	urinary volume
V	minute volume (of air or blood) visual acuity voice

$V_D V_T$	physiologic dead space in percent of tidal volume
V_E	airflow per unit of time
V_{Emax}	maximum flow per unit of time
V_P	plasma volume
V_T	tidal volume
$V\alpha$	alveolar ventilation visual acuity
VA	visual activity visual acuity
VALE	visual acuity, left eye
VARE	visual acuity, right eye
VC	acuity of color vision ventilatory capacity vital capacity
V/C	ventilation-circulation ratio
V_{CO_2}	carbon dioxide output
VDA	visual discriminatory acuity
VDV	ventricular end-diastolic volume
VF	vocal fremitus
VFP	ventricular fluid pressure
VIT CAP	vital capacity
V_{O_2}	oxygen consumption
VOD	vision, right eye
VOS	vision, left eye
VP	venous pressure
VR	vascular resistance venous return vocal resonance

VRBC	red blood cell volume
VRV	ventricular residual volume
VS	vital signs
VSW	ventricular stroke work
WHVP	wedged hepatic venous pressure
WRVP	wedged renal vein pressure
WV-MBC	ratio of walking ventilation to maximum breathing capacity

symptoms and diseases

AAA	abdominal aortic aneurysm
AAS	aortic arch syndrome
AB	asthmatic bronchitis
ABC	apnea, bradycardia, cyanosis
ABE	acute bacterial endocarditis
ABL	a-beta-lipoproteinemia
ACA	adenocarcinoma
ACC	adenoid cystic carcinoma
ACI	adrenal cortical insufficiency
ACVD	acute cardiovascular disease
ADEM	acute disseminated encephalomyelitis
ADS	antibody deficiency syndrome
AF	atrial fibrillation atrial flutter
AFI	amaurotic familial idiocy
AFIB	atrial fibrillation
AFL	atrial flutter
AGG	agammaglobulinemia

43

AGL acute granulocytic leukemia

AGN acute glomerulonephritis

AGS adrenogenital syndrome

AH amenorrhea and hirsutism
arterial hypertension
hypermetropic astigmatism

AHA acquired hemolytic anemia
autoimmune hemolytic anemia

AHD atherosclerotic heart disease
autoimmune hemolytic disease

AHLE acute hemorrhagic
leukoencephalitis

AI aortic insufficiency

AIHA autoimmune hemolytic anemia

AIP acute intermittent porphyria

ALD alcoholic liver disease

ALL acute lymphoblastic leukemia
acute lymphocytic leukemia
allergies

ALMI anterior lateral myocardial infarct

ALS amyotrophic lateral sclerosis

AM ametropia
anovular menstruation
myopic astigmatism

AMH mixed astigmatism with myopia
predominating

AMI acute myocardial infarction

AML	acute monocytic leukemia
	acute myeloblastic leukemia
	acute myelocytic leukemia
	acute myeloid leukemia
AMML	acute myelomonocytic leukemia
ANS	arteriolonephrosclerosis
AOD	arterial occlusive disease
AODM	adult onset diabetes mellitus
AOM	acute otitis media
AP	angina pectoris
APA	aldosterone-producing adenoma
APB	atrial premature beats
APC	atrial premature contractions
APH	antepartum hemorrhage
APL	accelerated painless labor
ARD	acute respiratory disease
ARF	acute respiratory failure
	acute rheumatic fever
AS	Adams-Stokes syndrome/disease
	ankylosing spondylitis
	aortic stenosis
	arteriosclerosis
ASCAD	arteriosclerotic coronary artery disease
ASCVD	arteriosclerotic cardiovascular disease
	atherosclerotic cardiovascular disease
ASD	aldosterone secretion defect
	atrial septal defect

ASH	hypermetropic astigmatism
ASHD	arteriosclerotic heart disease
ASHN	acute sclerosing hyaline necrosis
ASM	myopic astigmatism
ASMI	anteroseptal myocardial infarction
ASO	arteriosclerosis obliterans
AST	astigmatism
ATD	asphyxiating thoracic dystrophy
ATN	acute tubular necrosis
ATR FIB, At Fib	atrial fibrillation
ATS	anxiety tension state atherosclerosis
AUL	acute undifferentiated leukemia
AUR FIB	auricular fibrillation
AVH	acute viral hepatitis
AWI	anterior wall infarction
AWMI	anterior wall myocardial infarction
BA	bronchial asthma
BBB	bundle branch block
BBBB	bilateral bundle branch block
BCE	basal cell epithelioma
BE	bacterial endocarditis

BIH	benign intracranial hypertension
BN	brachial neuritis
BNO	bladder-neck obstruction
BOM	bilateral otitis media
BPD	bronchopulmonary dysplasia
BPH	benign prostatic hypertrophy
BSDLB	block in the anterosuperior division of the left branch
BT	bladder tumor brain tumor
BVH	biventricular hypertrophy
CA	cancer carcinoma cardiac arrest
CAD	coronary artery disease
CAG	chronic atrophic gastritis
CAH	chronic active hepatitis congenital adrenal hyperplasia
CAHD	coronary atherosclerotic heart disease
CAO	chronic airway obstruction
CAS	cerebral arteriosclerosis
CB	chronic bronchitis
CBA	chronic bronchitis with asthma
CBS	chronic brain syndrome
CCC	chronic calculous cholecystitis
CCE	cyanosis, clubbing, or edema
CCF	compound comminuted fracture congestive cardiac failure

CD	cardiovascular disease communicable disease contagious disease
CDH	congenital dislocation of hip
CE	cardiac enlargement clinical emphysema
CES	central excitatory state
CF	cardiac failure cystic fibrosis
CFP	cystic fibrosis of the pancreas
CG	chronic glomerulonephritis
CGD	chronic granulomatous disease
CGL	chronic granulocytic leukemia
CGN	chronic glomerulonephritis
CHA	congenital hypoplastic anemia
CHB	complete heart block
CHD	congenital heart disease coronary heart disease
CHF	congestive heart failure
CI	cardiac insufficiency cerebral infarction
CID	cytomegalic inclusion disease
CIDS	cellular immunity deficiency syndrome
CIN	central inhibitory state cervical intraepithelial neoplasia
CIS	carcinoma in situ
CL/CP	cleft lip and cleft palate
CLD	chronic liver disease chronic lung disease

CLE	centrilobular emphysema
CLL	chronic lymphatic leukemia chronic lymphocytic leukemia
CLSL	chronic lymphosarcoma (cell) leukemia
CM	chondromalacia
CMGN	chronic membranous glomerulonephritis
CMID	cytomegalic inclusion disease
CML	chronic myelocytic leukemia chronic myelogenous leukemia
CMM	cutaneous malignant melanoma
CMN	cystic medial necrosis
CMN-AA	cystic medial necrosis of the ascending aorta
CNE	chronic nervous exhaustion
CNHD	congenital nonspherocytic hemolytic disease
C of A	coarctation of aorta
COLD	chronic obstructive lung disease
COPD	chronic obstructive pulmonary disease
CP	cerebral palsy chronic pyelonephritis cleft palate cor pulmonale
CPE	chronic pulmonary emphysema
CPN	chronic pyelonephritis
CRD	chronic renal disease chronic respiratory disease

CRF	chronic renal failure
CRST	calcinosis cutis, Raynaud's phenomenon, sclerodactyly, and telangiectasis
CSH	chronic subdural hematoma cortical stromal hyperplasia
CSM	cerebrospinal meningitis
CT	cerebral thrombosis coronary thrombosis
CTS	carpal tunnel syndrome
CUC	chronic ulcerative colitis
CVA	cardiovascular accident cerebrovascular accident
CVAT	costovertebral angle tenderness
CVD	cardiovascular disease
CVH	combined ventricular hypertrophy
CWP	childbirth without pain
DA	degenerative arthritis
DAH	disordered action of the heart
DDD	degenerative disk disease
DDS	dystrophy-dystocia syndrome
DFU	dead fetus in utero
DH	delayed hypersensitivity
DI	diabetes insipidus
DIC	diffuse intravascular coagulation disseminated intravascular coagulation
DILD	diffuse infiltrative lung disease
DIP	desquamative interstitial pneumonia

DJD	degenerative joint disease
DKA	diabetic ketoacidosis
DLE	discoid lupus erythematosus
	disseminated lupus erythematosus
DM	diabetes mellitus
DMI	diaphragmatic myocardial infarct
DOE	dyspnea on exertion
DOPS	diffuse obstructive pulmonary syndrome
DPD	diffuse pulmonary disease
DS	Down's syndrome
DSAP	disseminated superficial actinic porokeratosis
DT	delirium tremens
DTP	distal tingling on percussion
DU	duodenal ulcer
DUB	dysfunctional uterine bleeding
DVT	deep venous thrombosis
E	emmetropia
EAC	Ehrlich ascites carcinoma
EAHF	eczema, asthma, hay fever
EEE	Eastern equine encephalitis
EFE	endocardial fibroelastosis
EGL	eosinophilic granuloma of the lung
EH	essential hypertension
EHC	essential hypercholesterolemia
EHL	endogenous hyperlipidemia
EHO	extrahepatic obstruction

EHPH	extrahepatic portal hypertension
EKC	epidemic keratoconjunctivitis
EM	emmetropia
EMC	encephalomyocarditis
EMF	endomyocardial fibrosis
EMG	exophthalmos, macroglossia, gigantism
EP	ectopic pregnancy
EPC	epilepsia partialis continua
FB	foreign body
FBD	functional bowel disorder
FC	finger clubbing
FECP	free erythrocyte coproporphyria
FF	flat feet
FGD	fatal granulomatous disease
FI	fever caused by infection
FJN	familial juvenile nephrophthisis
FLSA	follicular lymphosarcoma
FMD	foot-and-mouth disease
FMF	familial Mediterranean fever
Fract	fracture
FR BB	fracture of both bones
FTT	failure to thrive
FUB	functional uterine bleeding
FUO	fever of unknown origin
FX	fracture
GABHS	group A beta-hemolytic streptococcus

GC, gc	gonococcal
	gonococcus
GF	gastric fistula
GGE	general gland enlargement
GG or S	glands, goiter, or stiffness
GHD	growth hormone deficiency
GIP	giant cell interstitial pneumonia
GIS	gas in stomach
GN	glomerulonephritis
GP	general paresis
GPI	general paralysis of the insane
GSD	glycogen storage disease
GSE	gluten-sensitive enteropathy
GSW	gunshot wound
GU	gastric ulcer
	gonococcal urethritis
GVHR	graft-vs-host reaction
H	hypermetropia
HA	headache
	hemolytic anemia
	high anxiety
HAE	hereditary angioedema
HANE	hereditary angioneurotic edema
HAP	heredopathia atactica polyneuritiformis
HASCVD	hypertensive arteriosclerotic cardiovascular disease
HASHD	hypertensive arteriosclerotic heart disease

HB	heart block
HBP	high blood pressure
HCD	heavy chain disease
HCP	hereditary coproporphyria
HCVD	hypertensive cardiovascular disease
HD	heart disease Hodgkin's disease hydatid disease
HDN	hemolytic disease of the newborn
HDS	herniated disk syndrome
HF	hay fever heart failure hemorrhagic fever
HFI	hereditary fructose intolerance
HHA	hereditary hemolytic anemia
HHD	hypertensive heart disease
H + Hm	compound hypermetropic astigmatism
HHNK	hyperglycemic, hyperosmolar, nonketotic (coma)
HHT	hereditary hemorrhagic telangiectasia
HI	high impulsiveness
HIHA	high impulsiveness, high anxiety
HILA	high impulsiveness, low anxiety
HIT	hypertrophic infiltrative tendinitis
HL	hypermetropia, latent
HLP	hyperlipoproteinemia

HM	heart murmur
	hydatidiform mole
	manifest hypermetropia
HMD	hyaline membrane disease
HMSAS	hypertrophic muscular subaortic stenosis
HN	hereditary nephritis
HNP	herniated nucleus pulposus
HNSHA	hereditary nonspherocytic hemolytic anemia
HOCM	hypertrophic obstructive cardiomyopathy
HOOD	hereditary osteo-onychodysplasia
HPS	hypertrophic pyloric stenosis
HPT	hyperparathyroidism
HPVD	hypertensive pulmonary vascular disease
HS	hereditary spherocytosis
	herpes simplex
HSV	herpes simplex virus
HT	hypermetropia, total
	hypertension
	hyperthyroidism
HTHD	hypertensive heart disease
HTN	hypertension
HUS	hemolytic-uremic syndrome
HV	hyperventilation
HVD	hypertensive vascular disease
HVSD	hydrogen-detected ventricular septal defect

Hy	hypermetropia
HY	hysteria
hypo	hypochromia
HYS	hysteria
HZ	herpes zoster
IADHS	inappropriate antidiuretic hormone syndrome
IAHD	idiopathic acquired hemolytic disease
IASD	interatrial septal defect
IC	intermittent claudication irritable colon
ICA	intracranial aneurysm
ICT	inflammation of connective tissue
IDA	iron deficiency anemia
IDD	insulin-dependent diabetes mellitus
IDM	idiopathic disease of the myocardium
IDS	immunity deficiency state
IH	infectious hepatitis
IHBTD	incompatible hemolytic blood transfusion disease
IHC	idiopathic hypercalciuria
IHD	ischemic heart disease
IHO	idiopathic hypertrophic osteoarthropathy
IHP	idiopathic hypoparathyroidism
IHPH	intrahepatic portal hypertension

IHSS	idiopathic hypertrophic subaortic stenosis
IID	insulin-independent diabetes mellitus
ILD	ischemic limb disease
IM	infectious mononucleosis
IMB	intermenstrual bleeding
IMH	idiopathic myocardial hypertrophy
INAD	infantile neuroaxonal dystrophy
INE	infantile necrotizing encephalomyelopathy
INF	infectious disease
INS	idiopathic nephrotic syndrome
IO	intestinal obstruction
IOFB	intraocular foreign body
IPH	idiopathic pulmonary hemosiderosis
IRBBB	incomplete right bundle branch block
IRDS	idiopathic respiratory distress syndrome
ISH	icteric serum hepatitis
ITP	idiopathic thrombocytopenic purpura
IUFB	intrauterine foreign body
IUM	intrauterine fetally malnourished
IVCC	intravascular consumption coagulopathy
IVCD	intraventricular conduction defect
IVH	intraventricular hemorrhage

IVSD	interventricular septal defect
IWMI	inferior wall myocardial infarction
JBE	Japanese B encephalitis
JODM	juvenile onset diabetes mellitus
JRA	juvenile rheumatoid arthritis
KA	ketoacidosis
KCS	keratoconjunctivitis sicca
KW	Kimmelstiel-Wilson syndrome
LA	low anxiety
lac	laceration
LAE	left atrial enlargement
LAH	left atrial hypertrophy
LBBB	left bundle branch block
LBP	low back pain
LBW	low birth weight
LBWI	low-birth-weight infant
LC	Laennec's cirrhosis
LCL	lymphocytic lymphosarcoma
LCM	lymphatic choriomeningitis
	lymphocytic choriomeningitis
LE	lupus erythematosus
LED	lupus erythematosus disseminatus
LES	systemic lupus erythematosus
LGN	lobular glomerulonephritis
LHF	left heart failure
LIAFI	late infantile amaurotic familial idiocy
LIHA	low impulsiveness, high anxiety

LILA	low impulsiveness, low anxiety
LLC	lymphocytic leukemia, chronic
LMNL	lower motor neuron lesion
LN	lipoid nephrosis lupus nephritis
LOS	low output syndrome
LOWBI	low-birth-weight infant
LPV	lymphopathia venereum
LS	lymphosarcoma
LSA/RCS	lymphosarcoma-reticulum cell sarcoma
LTB	laryngotracheobronchitis
LVE	left ventricular enlargement
LVF	left ventricular failure
LVH	left ventricular hypertrophy
LVI	left ventricular insufficiency
LW	lacerating wound
M	myopia
(m)	murmur
M + Am	myopic astigmatism
MAP	megaloblastic anemia of pregnancy
MBD	minimal brain dysfunction
MC	myocarditis
MCD	medullary cystic disease
MD	manic-depressive muscular dystrophy myocardial disease
MDI	manic-depressive illness

MDUO	myocardial disease of unknown origin
MEA	multiple endocrine adenomatosis
MF	mycosis fungoides
MFW	multiple fragment wounds
MG	myasthenia gravis
MGN	membranous glomerulonephritis
MHA	microangiopathic hemolytic anemia
MHN	massive hepatic necrosis
MI	mitral insufficiency myocardial infarction
MLA	monocytic leukemia, acute
MLC	myelomonocytic leukemia, chronic
MLD	metachromatic leukodystrophy
MLS	myelomonocytic leukemia, subacute
MM	malignant melanoma multiple myeloma myeloid metaplasia
MMM	myeloid metaplasia with myelofibrosis myelosclerosis with myeloid metaplasia
MODM	mature onset diabetes mellitus
Mono	infectious mononucleosis
MPGN	mesangioproliferative glomerulonephritis

MR	mental retardation
	mitral reflux
	mitral regurgitation
MS	multiple sclerosis
MS, ms	mitral stenosis
MSUD	maple syrup urine disease
MT	malignant teratoma
MTI	malignant teratoma intermediate
MTT	malignant teratoma trophoblastic
MVE	Murray Valley encephalitis
My	myopia
MyG	myasthenia gravis
NBTE	nonbacterial thrombotic endocarditis
NCA	neurocirculatory asthenia
NCNCA	normochromic normocytic anemia
ND	neurotic depression
NDI	nephrogenic diabetes insipidus
NEC	necrotizing enterocolitis
NGU	nongonococcal urethritis
NHA	nonspecific hepatocellular abnormality
NND	neonatal death
noc	nocturia
NPC	nodal premature contractions
NPCa	nasopharyngeal carcinoma
NPDR	nonproliferative diabetic retinopathy
NS	nephrotic syndrome

NSU	nonspecific urethritis
NTG	nontoxic goiter
NTN	nephrotoxic nephritis
N&V	nausea and vomiting
NVD	nausea, vomiting, and diarrhea nonvalvular (heart) disease
OA	osteoarthritis
OAD	obstructive airway disease
OAP	osteoarthropathy
OBS	organic brain syndrome
OF	osteitis fibrosa
OM	otitis media osteomalacia
OMCA	acute catarrhal otitis media
OMD	ocular muscle dystrophy
OMI	old myocardial infarction
OMPA	acute purulent otitis media
OS, os	osteosclerosis
osteo	osteomyelitis
P	presbyopia
PA	paralysis agitans pernicious anemia primary amenorrhea primary anemia
PAC	premature atrial contraction premature auricular contraction
PAF	pulmonary arteriovenous fistula
PAFIB	paroxysmal atrial fibrillation
PAH	pulmonary artery hypertension

PAM	pulmonary alveolar microlithiasis
PAN	periarteritis nodosa
PAOD	peripheral arterial occlusive disease
PAP	primary atypical pneumonia pulmonary alveolar proteinosis
PAS	pulmonary artery stenosis
PAT	paroxysmal atrial tachycardia
PBC	primary biliary cirrhosis
PBN	paralytic brachial neuritis
PCD	polycystic disease
PCH	paroxysmal cold hemoglobinuria
PCM	protein-calorie malnutrition
PCV	polycythemia vera
PCV-M	myeloid metaplasia with polycythemia vera
PD	Parkinson's disease psychotic depression pulmonary disease
PE	pleural effusion pulmonary edema pulmonary embolism
PEO	progressive external ophthalmoplegia
PET	preeclamptic toxemia
PFT	posterior fossa tumor
PH	prostatic hypertrophy pulmonary hypertension
PHP	primary hyperparathyroidism pseudohypoparathyroidism

PI	pulmonary infarction
PID	pelvic inflammatory disease
PIE	pulmonary infiltration with eosinophilia
	pulmonary interstitial emphysema
PKU	phenylketonuria
PLD	platelet defect
PM	polymyositis
	presystolic murmur
PMA	progressive muscular atrophy
PMD	primary myocardial disease
	progressive muscular dystrophy
PMI	posterior myocardial infarction
PML	progressive multifocal leukoencephalopathy
PMS	postmenopausal syndrome
PN	periarteritis nodosa
	peripheral neuropathy
	pneumonia
	psychoneurotic
	pyelonephritis
PND	paroxysmal nocturnal dyspnea
PND, pnd	postnasal drip
pneu	pneumonia
PNH	paroxysmal nocturnal hemoglobinuria
POA	primary optic atrophy
poik	poikilocytosis
PPD	permanent partial disability

PPH	primary pulmonary hypertension
	postpartum hemorrhage
PPS	postperfusion syndrome
PR	presbyopia
PS	pulmonary stenosis
	pyloric stenosis
PSC	posterior subcapsular cataract
PSE	portal-systemic encephalopathy
PSGN	poststreptococcal glomerulonephritis
PSS	progressive systemic sclerosis
PT	pneumothorax
	paroxysmal tachycardia
PTA	post-traumatic amnesia
PTC	pheochromocytoma, thyroid carcinoma syndrome
PTD	permanent total disability
PTE	pulmonary thromboembolism
PTH	post-transfusion hepatitis
PTI	persistent tolerant infection
PTM	post-transfusion mononucleosis
PU	peptic ulcer
PUD	pulmonary disease
PUO	pyrexia of unknown origin
PV	polycythemia vera
PVC	premature ventricular contraction
	pulmonary venous congestion
PVD	peripheral vascular disease
PVT	paroxysmal ventricular tachycardia
	portal vein thrombosis

PWI	posterior wall infarct
PX	pneumothorax
RA	rheumatoid arthritis
RAD	reactive airway disease
RAE	right atrial enlargement
RAH	right atrial hypertrophy
RAS	renal artery stenosis
RBBB	right bundle branch block
RCS	reticulum cell sarcoma
RD	Raynaud's disease respiratory disease retinal detachment
RDS	respiratory distress syndrome
RE	regional enteritis
RF	rheumatic fever
RHD	rheumatic heart disease
RHF	right heart failure
RI	regional ileitis respiratory illness
RIOJ	recurrent intrahepatic obstructive jaundice
RKW	renal potassium wasting
RLF	retrolental fibroplasia
RMSF	Rocky Mountain spotted fever
ROM	rupture of membranes
RPGN	rapidly progressive glomerulonephritis
RS	Reiter's syndrome
RSA	reticulum cell sarcoma

RSS	Russian spring-summer (encephalitis)
RTA	renal tubular acidosis
RURTI	recurrent upper respiratory tract infection
RVE	right ventricular enlargement
RVH	right ventricular hypertrophy
RVT	renal vein thrombosis
SA	sarcoma secondary amenorrhea secondary anemia
SAA	Stokes-Adams attacks
SAB	significant asymptomatic bacteriuria subarachnoid block
SACD	subacute combined degeneration
SAH	subarachnoid hemorrhage
SAS	supravalvular aortic stenosis
SB	sinus bradycardia stillbirth
SBE	subacute bacterial endocarditis
SBO	small bowel obstruction
SBS	social-breakdown syndrome
SCC	squamous cell carcinoma
SD	septal defect shoulder disarticulation spontaneous delivery sudden death
SDH	subdural hematoma
SDS	sensory deprivation syndrome sudden death syndrome

SED	spondyloepiphyseal dysplasia
SEMI	subendocardial myocardial injury, infarction
SFW	shrapnel fragment wound
SH	serum hepatitis sinus histiocytosis
SHO	secondary hypertrophic osteoarthropathy
SHP	surgical hypoparathyroidism
SIADH	syndrome of inappropriate antidiuretic hormone
SIDS	sudden infant death syndrome
SIW	self-inflicted wound
SLE	systemic lupus erythematosus
SLKC	superior limbic keratoconjunctivitis
SM	systolic murmur
SMON	subacute myelo-optical neuropathy
SNHL	sensorineural hearing loss
SOB	shortness of breath
SOM	secretory otitis media serous otitis media
Sq cell ca	squamous cell carcinoma
SS	sickle cell anemia Sjögren's syndrome subaortic stenosis
SSPE	subacute sclerosing panencephalitis
SSS	sick sinus syndrome

ST	sinus tachycardia
Still B	stillborn
SUD	sudden unexpected death sudden unexplained death
SUID	sudden unexplained infant death
SUUD	sudden unexpected unexplained death
SVAS	supravalvular aortic stenosis
SVD	spontaneous vaginal delivery spontaneous vertex delivery
SW	stab wound
syph	syphilis
Sz	seizure
SZ	schizophrenia
T	tumor
TAD	thoracic asphyxiant dystrophy
TAL	thymic alymphoplasia
TAO	thromboangiitis obliterans
TAR	thrombocytopenia with absence of the radius
TB	tracheobronchitis tuberculosis
TBC, tbc	tuberculosis
TBM	tuberculous meningitis
TB-RD	tuberculosis-respiratory disease
TCI	transient cerebral ischemia
TD	total disability
TDF	thoracic duct fistula
TE	tetanus

TEF	tracheoesophageal fistula
TFS	testicular feminization syndrome
TG	toxic goiter
TGAR	total graft area rejected
thromb	thrombosis
TI	tricuspid incompetence
	tricuspid insufficiency
TIA	transient ischemic attack
TIE	transient ischemic episode
TIS	tumor in situ
TNM	tumor, nodes, metastases
T of A	transposition of aorta
TOA	tubo-ovarian abscess
TP	thrombocytopenic purpura
TPH	transplacental hemorrhage
TRIC	trachoma inclusion conjunctivitis
TS	tricuspid stenosis
TSD	Tay-Sachs disease
TSS	toxic shock syndrome
	tropical splenomegaly syndrome
TTP	thrombotic thrombocytopenic purpura
TV	*Trichomonas* vaginitis
UC	ulcerative colitis
UCD	usual childhood diseases
UCS	unconscious
UD	urethral discharge
UPI	uteroplacental insufficiency

URD	upper respiratory disease
URI	upper respiratory infection
URTI	upper respiratory tract infection
UTI	urinary tract infection
VD	venereal disease
VDG	venereal disease—gonorrhea
VDH	valvular disease of the heart
VDS	venereal disease—syphilis
VEE	Venezuelan equine encephalitis
VF	ventricular fibrillation
VH	viral hepatitis
VHD	valvular heart disease viral hematodepressive disease
VRI	viral respiratory infection
VS	villonodular synovitis
VSD	ventricular septal defect
VT	ventricular tachycardia
VV	varicose veins
WC	whooping cough
WE	Western encephalitis Western encephalomyelitis
WEE	Western equine encephalomyelitis
WPW	Wolff-Parkinson-White syndrome
YF	yellow fever
ZE	Zollinger-Ellison syndrome

diagnostic terms

ABC	absolute basophil count
ABG, ABGs	arterial blood gas arterial blood gases
ACG	angiocardiography apexcardiogram
ACT	activated coagulation time anticoagulant therapy
AEG	air encephalogram
AGT	antiglobulin test
AGTT	abnormal glucose tolerance test
AHT	augmented histamine test
AMH	automated medical history
AMS	automated multiphasic screening
ANAL	analysis analyst
ANG	angiogram
angio	angiography
A&P	auscultation and palpation
APTT	activated partial thromboplastin time
ART	Achilles tendon reflex test

ATT	aspirin tolerance time
Au(1)	Australia antigen
AUSC	auscultation
aVR, aVF, aVL	augmented unipolar ECG leads
AVT	Allen vision test
AZT, AZ test	Aschheim-Zondek pregnancy test
BaEn	barium enema
BALB	binaural alternate loudness balance test
BAP	blood agar plate
BB	breast biopsy
BCG	ballistocardiogram bicolor guaiac test
BDE	bile duct exploration
BE	barium enema
BFP	biologic false positive
BFT	bentonite flocculation test
BG	Bordet Gengou test
BGlu	blood glucose
BGTT	borderline glucose tolerance test
bl cult	blood culture
BLT	blood clot lysis time
BNPA	binasal pharyngeal airway
BSP	Bromsulphalein test (liver function)
BT	bleeding time

BUN	blood urea nitrogen
BX, Bx	biopsy
C_{alb}, **C.alb.**	albumin clearance
C_{CR}, C_{Cr}, C_{cr}	creatinine clearance
C_{in}	insulin clearance
C_u	urea clearance
CAT	Children's Apperception Test computerized axial tomography
CATH, Cath	catheter catheterization catheterize
CBC	complete blood count
CC	creatinine clearance
CCAT	conglutinating complement absorption test
CCMSU	clean catch midstream urine
C.Cr.	creatinine clearance
C&D	cystoscopy and dilatation
CD_{50}	median curative dose
CDE	common duct exploration
CEPH-FLOC	cephalin flocculation test
CFF	critical flicker fusion test
CFT	complement fixation test
CGTT	cortisone-glucose tolerance test
CICU	coronary intensive care unit
CLT	clot lysis time

CMG	cystometrogram
COGTT	cortisone-primed oral glucose tolerance test
CORA	conditioned orientation reflex audiometry
CR	colon resection
CRO	cathode ray oscillograph
C&S	culture and sensitivity
CT	circulation time
	clotting time
	computerized tomography
	Coombs' test
	corneal transplant
	corrective therapy
CTA	cytotoxic assay
CT scan	computerized tomography scan
CUG	cystourethrogram
CVS	clean-voided specimen
CX, CXR	chest X-ray
Cysto	cystoscopy
DAP	direct agglutination pregnancy test
	Draw-a-Person Test
DAPT	direct agglutination pregnancy test
DBCL	dilute blood clot lysis (method)
DC	dilatation and curettage
	direct Coombs' test
D&C	dilatation and curettage
DCT	direct Coombs' test

D&E	dilation and evacuation
Diag	diagnosis
Diff	differential blood count differential leukocyte count
DL	Donath-Landsteiner test
DPG	displacement placentogram
DST	dexamethasone suppression test
DT	distance test
Dx	diagnosis
EBL	estimated blood loss
E/C	endo/cystoscopy
ECG	electrocardiogram
ECHO	echocardiogram
ECLT	euglobulin clot lysis time
ED	effective dose
ED_{50}	median effective dose
EDD	effective drug duration
EDR	effective direct radiation
EEA	electroencephalic audiometry
EEG	electroencephalogram
EGG	electrogastrogram
EGM	electrogram
EKG	electrocardiogram
EKY	electrokymogram
ELT	euglobulin lysis time
EMG	electromyelography electromyogram electromyography

EN	enema
ENEM	enema
ENG	electronystagmogram electronystagmograph
EOG	electro-oculogram
ERA	evoked response audiometry
ERG	electroretinogram
ESO	esophagoscopy
ETT	exercise tolerance test
Ex	examination
FA	first aid
FAT	fluorescent antibody test
FBE	full blood examination
FBS	fasting blood sugar
FD	fatal dose
FD_{50}	median fatal dose
FECG, FEKG	fetal electrocardiogram
FES	forced expiratory spirogram
FH, FH_x	family history
FIT	fusion inferred threshold test
fluoro	fluoroscopy
Fried. test	Friedman test (pregnancy)
FS	frozen section

FTA-AB,
  FTA-ABS
	fluorescent treponemal
	  antibody absorption test

FVL	femoral vein ligation
FW	Felix-Weil reaction Folin and Wu's (method)

FWR	Felix-Weil reaction
FX	fluoroscopy frozen section
F-Y test	fibrinogen, qualitative test
GA	gastric analysis general anesthesia
GITT	glucose-insulin tolerance test
GTT	glucose tolerance test
GXT	graded exercise test
GZ	Guilford-Zimmerman personality test
HEAT	human erythrocyte agglutination test
HED	unit of roentgen-ray dosage (*Haut-Einheits-Dosis*)
HIT	hemagglutination-inhibition test
H&P	history and physical
HPE	history and physical examination
HPI	history of present illness
HRE	high-resolution electrocardiogram
HSG	hysterosalpingogram
HTP	House-Tree-Person test
Hx	history
HYPO	injection (hypodermic)
IAE	intra-atrial electrocardiogram
IAS	intra-amniotic saline infusion
IAT	invasive activity test iodine-azide test
ICT	indirect Coombs' test

ID	ineffective dose
IDP	initial dose period
IDVC	indwelling venous catheter
IEMG	integrated electromyogram
IEOP	immunoelectro-osmophoresis
IEP	immunoelectrophoresis
IFRA	indirect fluorescent rabies antibody test
IHO	idiopathic hypertrophic osteoarthropathy
IHT	intravenous histamine test
IMI	intramuscular injection
INF, Inf	infusion
INJ	inject
INOC	inoculate
IPG	impedance plethysmography
IPPB	intermittent positive pressure breathing
IPPO	intermittent positive pressure inflation with oxygen
IPPR	intermittent positive pressure respiration
IPPV	intermittent positive pressure ventilation
IPRT	interpersonal reaction test
IRS	infrared spectrophotometry
IST	insulin sensitivity test

IT	implantation test
	inhalation test
	intradermal test
	intratracheal tube
ITPA	Illinois Test of Psycholinguistic Abilities
ITT	insulin tolerance test
IVC	intravenous cholangiogram
IVCV	inferior venacavography
IVGTT	intravenous glucose tolerance test
IVP	intravenous pyelogram
IVTTT	intravenous tolbutamide tolerance test
IVU	intravenous urography
KCG	kinetocardiogram
KPTT	kaolin partial thromboplastin time
KRP	Kolmer's test with Reiter protein
KS	Kveim-Siltzbach test
KW	Keith-Wagener test
L&A	light and accommodation (pupil reaction)
LA	local anesthesia
LAG	lymphangiogram
LAIT	latex agglutination inhibition test
Lam	laminogram
lap	laparotomy
LD	laboratory data
LFD	lactose-free diet

LFT	latex flocculation test
	liver function test
LOC	level of consciousness
LP	lumbar puncture
LPE	lipoprotein electrophoresis
LTT	lymphoblastic transformation test
MAS	Manifest Anxiety Scale
MED	minimal erythema dose
MFD	minimal fatal dose
MFT	muscle function test
MH	marital history
MH, M Hx	medical history
MICU	mobile intensive care unit
MIRD	medical internal radiation dose
MIRU	myocardial infarction research unit
MLD	minimum lethal dose
MMPI	Minnesota Multiphasic Personality Inventory
MMR	mass miniature radiography
	mobile mass X-ray
MPD	maximum permissible dose
MPI	multiphasic personality inventory
MRD	minimum reacting dose
MRT	milk-ring test
MSRPP	multidimensional scale for rating psychiatric patients
MSS	mental status schedule
MTD	maximum tolerated dose

MTDT	modified tone decay test
NLT	normal lymphocyte transfer test
NNN	Nicolle-Novy-MacNeal (medium)
NPT	neoprecipitin test
NST	nonstress test
NT	neutralization test
OBP	ova, blood, and parasites (stool exam)
OCG	oral cholecystogram
ODM	ophthalmodynamometry
O&E	observation and examination
OGTT	oral glucose tolerance test
OH	occupational history
OSM	oxygen saturation meter
OST	object sorting test
OT	objective test
OU	Observation Unit
P&A	percussion and auscultation
palp	palpate, palpated, palpable
PAP, Pap	Papanicolaou (smear, stain, test)
PAS	periodic acid-Schiff (method, stain, technique, test)
PCA	percutaneous carotid arteriogram
PCG	phonocardiogram
PCT	plasmacrit test
PE	physical evaluation physical examination

PEG	pneumoencephalogram
PEP	Psychiatric Evaluation Profile
PERL	pupils equal and reactive to light
PERLA	pupils equal, react to light and accommodation
PERRLA	pupils equal, round, react to light and accommodation
PEx	physical examination
PF	picture-frustration (study)
PFQ	personality factor questionnaire
PFT	pulmonary function test
PH	personal history
PH, P Hx	past history
PI	present illness
PIP	Psychotic Inpatient Profile
PIT	patellar inhibition test
PL	placebo
PMA	Primary Mental Abilities test
PMH	past medical history
PMT	Porteus maze test
P&P	prothrombin and proconvertin test
PRERLA	pupils round, equal, react to light and accommodation
procto	proctoscopy
pro-time	prothrombin time
PRP	Psychotic Reaction Profile
PS	prescription

PSP	phenolsulfonphthalein test
PT	prothrombin time
PTT, Ptt	partial thromboplastin time
PX	physical examination
QMT	quantitative muscle testing
Qt	Quick's test
QUICHA	quantitative inhalation challenge apparatus
R	Rinne test
RAIU	radioactive iodine uptake
RBC	red blood cell count red blood count
RBS	random blood sugar
RCC	red cell count
REG	radioencephalogram
REP	retrograde pyelogram
RF	rheumatoid factor
RFS	renal function study
RFT	rod-and-frame test
Rh	Rhesus blood factor
RIA	radioimmunoassay
RIU	radioactive iodine uptake
RKY	roentgen kymography
RP	retrograde pyelogram
RPCF, RPCFT	Reiter protein complement fixation test
RPG	retrograde pyelogram
RPR	rapid plasma reagin test

RR&E, RRE	round, regular, and equal (pupils)
RST	radiosensitivity test
RT	reading test respiratory therapy
Rx	prescription treatment
S/A	sugar/acetone (urine)
SB	Stanford-Binet test
SB_{N2}	single-breath nitrogen test
SBT	single-breath test
SC	sickle cell test
SCAT	sheep cell agglutination test
SCT	sex chromatin test staphylococcal clumping test
SEA test	sheep erythrocyte agglutination test
Sed rate	sedimentation rate
SEG	sonoencephalogram
SG test	Sachs-Georgi test
SHT	subcutaneous histamine test
Sigmoid	sigmoidoscopy
SISI	short increment sensitivity index (hearing test)
SMA-12	12-channel biochemical profile (sequential multiple analysis)
SNB	scalene node biopsy
SRFS	split renal function study
SRT	speech reception test

SSA	sulfosalicylic acid test
SSE	soapsuds enema
STS	serologic test for syphilis
	standard test for syphilis
STT	serial thrombin time
STYCAR	Screening Tests for Young Children and Retardates
SVCG	spatial vectorcardiogram
SW	Schwartz-Watson test
Sx	symptoms
TAT	thematic apperception test
	thromboplastin activation test
TATST	tetanus antitoxin skin test
TC	throat culture
	tissue culture
TCD	tissue culture dose
TCID	tissue culture infective dose
TCM	tissue culture medium
TCT	thrombin clotting time
TDT	tone decay test
TEG	thromboelastogram
TGT	thromboplastin generation time
THER	therapy
TIT	*Treponema* immobilization test
TKD	tokodynamometer
TKG	tokodynagraph
TLA	translumbar aortogram
TLC	thin-layer chromatography

TLD	thermoluminescent dosimeter
TMAS	Taylor Manifest Anxiety Scale
TNI	total nodal irradiation
TOWER	testing, orientation, work, evaluation, rehabilitation
TPCF	*Treponema pallidum* complement-fixation test
TPI	treponemal immobilization (test) *Treponema pallidum* immobilization test
TRAM	Treatment Rating Assessment Matrix Treatment Response Assessment Method
TST	tumor skin test
TT	thrombin time
TTT	tolbutamide tolerance test
UA, U/A	urinalysis
UA	uterine aspiration
UBI	ultraviolet blood irradiation
UC	urethral catheterization
U/C	urine culture
USR	unheated serum reagin test
UVR	ultraviolet radiation
VA	vacuum aspiration
VASC	Verbal Auditory Screen for Children
VCG	vectorcardiogram
VDRL	Venereal Disease Research Laboratory test for syphilis

VDRS	Verdun Depression Rating Scale
VIS	vaginal irrigation smear
VP	venipuncture
V/Q Scan	ventilation perfusion of lung scan
VTSRS	Verdun Target Symptom Rating Scale
W	Weber's test
WAIS	Wechsler Adult Intelligence Scale
WBC	white blood cell count white blood count
WCC	white cell count
WFR	Weil-Felix reaction
WISC	Wechsler Intelligence Scale for Children
WPRS	Wittenborn Psychiatric Rating Scale
WR	Wassermann reaction
XR	X-ray
Zn fl	zinc flocculation test

therapeutic terms

ab	abortion
ABD HYST	abdominal hysterectomy
ACR	anticonstipation regimen
ACT	anticoagulation therapy
AH	abdominal hysterectomy
AKA	above-knee amputation
AK amp	above-knee amputation
alcr	alcohol rub
AMP	amputation
A-P	abdominal-perineal (resection)
APPY	appendectomy
AR	artificial respiration
ARD	anorectal dressing
AVR	aortic valve replacement
AVS	arteriovenous shunt
BG	bone graft
BKA	below-knee amputation
BNPA	binasal pharyngeal airway
BSO	bilateral sagittal osteotomy bilateral salpingo-oophorectomy

BSS	black silk suture
CABG	coronary artery bypass graft
CAS	cardiac surgery
CATH, cath	catheter catheterization catheterize
CCU	coronary care unit
CICU	cardiology intensive care unit coronary intensive care unit
Circ	circumcision
CNH	community nursing home
CPB	cardiopulmonary bypass
CR	colon resection
CRS	colon-rectal surgery
CS	cesarean section
CST	convulsive shock therapy
CT	corneal transplant corrective therapy
CU	convalescent unit
CVS	cardiovascular surgery
DC	dilatation and curettage
D&C	dilatation and curettage
DD	dry dressing
D&E	dilation and evacuation
DXT	deep X-ray therapy
ECF	extended care facility
ECS	electroconvulsive shock
ECT	electroconvulsive therapy

EDR	effective direct radiation
EG	esophagogastrectomy
EN, ENEM	enema
EST	electroshock therapy
FA	first aid
FD	forceps delivery
FTG	full-thickness graft
FVL	femoral vein ligation
GA	general anesthesia
GE	gastroenterostomy
GR	gastric resection
GT	gingiva, treatment of
HD	hemodialysis
HED	unit of roentgen-ray dosage *(Haut-Einheits-Dosis)*
HLR	heart-lung resuscitator
HMP	hot moist packs
H&R	hysterectomy and radiation
H&V	hemigastrectomy and vagotomy
HYPO, Hypo	injection (hypodermic)
Hyst, hyst	hysterectomy
IABP	intra-aortic balloon pump
IAS	intra-amniotic saline infusion
IC	intensive care
ICC	intensive coronary care
ICCU	intensive coronary care unit
ICF	intensive care facility

ICT	insulin coma therapy insulin convulsive therapy
ICU	intensive care unit
I&D	incision and drainage
IDVC	indwelling venous catheter
IMF	intermaxillary fixation
IMI	intramuscular injection
IMV	intermittent mandatory ventilation
INF	infusion
INJ	inject
INOC	inoculate
INPV	intermittent negative-pressure assisted ventilation
IOU	intensive therapy observation unit
IPPB	intermittent positive-pressure breathing
IPPI	interruption of pregnancy for psychiatric indication
IPPO	intermittent positive pressure inflation with oxygen
IPPR	intermittent positive pressure respiration
IPPV	intermittent positive pressure ventilation
IRR	irradiation
IST	insulin shock therapy
IT	inhalation therapy intensive therapy intratracheal tube
ITU	intensive therapy unit

IUT	intrauterine transfusion
IVPB	intravenous piggyback
IVT	intravenous transfusion
LA	local anesthesia
lam	laminectomy
LFD	lactose-free diet
	low forceps delivery
LG	laryngectomy
LLB	long leg brace
LLC	long leg cast
LME	left mediolateral episiotomy
LRM	left radical mastectomy
LSCS	lower segment cesarean section
LX	local irradiation
MA, MA tube	Miller-Abbott tube
MANIP	manipulation
MCCU	mobile coronary care unit
MEDS	medications
	medicines
MFD	midforceps delivery
MICU	medical intensive care unit
	mobile intensive care unit
MT	maximal therapy
	music therapy
NNR	New and Nonofficial Remedies
NS	neurosurgery
OBS	obstetrical service

Occup Rx	occupational therapy
oint	ointment
OP, op	operation
OPC	outpatient clinic
OPD	outpatient department
OPS	outpatient service
OPT	outpatient treatment
OR	operating room
ORS	orthopedic surgery
OS	oral surgery
OT	occupational therapy
OU	observation unit
PAR	postanesthesia room
PB	pressure breathing
PCB	paracervical block
PD	postural drainage
PEEP, Peep	positive end-expiratory pressure
PICU	pulmonary intensive care unit
PL	placebo
PPM	permanent pacemaker
PS	plastic surgery prescription
PT	physical therapy
PTX	parathyroidectomy
P&V	pyloroplasty and vagotomy
QAP	quinine, Atabrine, Plasmoquine (treatment)

RCU	respiratory care unit
Rehab	rehabilitation
RHB	right heart bypass
RICU	respiratory intensive care unit
RM	radical mastectomy
RND	radical neck dissection
RT	radiation therapy respiratory therapy
Rx	prescription treatment
S	surgery
SG	skin graft
SLR	straight leg raising
SM	simple mastectomy
SMR	submucous resection
SO	salpingo-oophorectomy
SPP	suprapubic prostatectomy
SSE	soapsuds enema
STSG	split-thickness skin graft
Supp	suppository
SVC-RPA shunt	superior vena cava-right pulmonary artery shunt
SVG	saphenous vein graft
TA	therapeutic abortion
T&A	tonsillectomy and adenoidectomy
TAB	therapeutic abortion

TAH	total abdominal hysterectomy
	transabdominal hysterectomy
TAHBSO	total abdominal hysterectomy, bilateral salpingo-oophorectomy
TCB	total cardiopulmonary bypass
TCP	therapeutic continuous penicillin
TDI	total-dose infusion
TEP	thromboendophlebectomy
THER, Ther	therapy
Thor	thoracic surgery
THR	total hip replacement
TKR	total knee replacement
TL	tubal ligation
TNI	total nodal irradiation
TPM	temporary pacemaker
TPN	total parenteral nutrition
T-PTX	thyroparathyroidectomy
TQ	tourniquet
Trach	tracheostomy
tract	traction
trt	treatment
TS	thoracic surgery
TUR	transurethral resection
TURB	transurethral resection of the bladder
TURBT	transurethral resection of bladder tumor

TURP	transurethral resection of the prostate
TVH	total vaginal hysterectomy
TX	traction transplant treatment
UBI	ultraviolet blood irradiation
UC	urethral catheterization
US	ultrasound
USO	unilateral salpingo-oophorectomy
VAG HYST	vaginal hysterectomy
VH	vaginal hysterectomy
V&P	vagotomy and pyloroplasty
VR	vocational rehabilitation
VR&E	vocational rehabilitation and education
VS	venisection
WBR	whole body radiation

orders/
instructions

$\overline{a}$	before *(ante)*
A	water *(aqua)*
AA, aa	of each *(ana)*
A&A	aid and attendance
abs	absent, away from

ABS FEB,
  abs feb
	while the fever is absent
	    (absente febre)

AC, ac	before meals *(ante cibum)*
ADD, add	let there be added *(adde)* average daily dose

AD DEF AN,
  ad def an
	to the point of fainting
	    (ad defectionem animi)

AD GRAT ACID,
  ad grat acid
	to an agreeable sourness
	    (ad gratum aciditatem)

ADHIB, adhib	to be administered *(adhibendus)*
Ad hoc	for this, temporary
ADL	activities of daily living
AD LIB, ad lib	as desired *(ad libitum)*

ADMOV,
  admov
	add, let there be added
	    (admove, admoveatur)

AD POND OM,
ad pond om
to the weight of the whole *(ad pondus omnium)*

ADT
anything desired

AD 2 VIC,
ad 2 vic
for two doses *(ad duas vices)*

ADV, adv
against *(adversum)*

AEG, aeg
the patient *(aeger, aegra)*

AGGRED FEB,
aggred feb
while the fever is coming on *(aggrediente febre)*

AGIT
shake *(agita)*

AGIT VAS,
agit vas
the vial being shaken *(agitato vase)*

alt
alternate

alt die, ALT DIEB,
alt dieb
alternate days, every other day *(alternis diebus)*

ALT HOR,
alt hor
every other hour *(alternis horis)*

ALT NOC,
alt noc
every other night *(alternis noctibus)*

ALV ADST,
alv adst
when the bowels are constipated *(alvo adstricta)*

AMA
against medical advice

ana
so much of each

ANTE, ante
before

AQ, aq
water *(aqua)*

Aq
aqueous

AQ BULL, **aq bull**	boiling water *(aqua bulliens)*
AQ DEST, **aq dest**	distilled water *(aqua destillata)*
AQ DIST, **aq dist**	distilled water
AQ FERV, **aq ferv**	hot water *(aqua fervens)*
AQ FRIG, **aq frig**	cold water *(aqua frigida)*
AQ PUR, **aq pur**	pure water *(aqua pura)*
AQ TEP, **aq tep**	tepid water *(aqua tepida)*
B, b	bath
BAL, bal	bath *(balneum)*
BD	base of prism down twice a day *(bis die)*
BI	base of prism in
BIB, bib	drink *(bibe)*
BID, bid	twice a day *(bis in die)*
BIN, bin	twice a night *(bis in nocte)*
BIS, bis	twice
BM	sea-water bath *(balneum maris)*
BO	base of prism out
BOL, bol	pill *(bolus)*
BR	bedrest
BRP	bathroom privileges
BU	base of prism up

BULL, bull	let it boil *(bulliat)*
BV	vapor bath *(balneum vaporis)*
c, c̄	with *(cum)*
CALEF, calef	warmed *(calefactus)*
CAP, cap	capsule let him take *(capiat)*
CC	chief complaint
CCW	counterclockwise
CDC	calculated date of confinement
cf	compare, refer to
CF	compare count fingers
CIB, cib	food *(cibus)*
CM	tomorrow morning *(cras mane)*
CMS, cms	to be taken tomorrow morning *(cras mane sumendus)*
CN	tomorrow night *(cras nocte)*
CNS, cns	to be taken tomorrow night *(cras nocte sumendus)*
C/O	complains of
COCHL, cochl	spoonful *(cochleare)*
COCHL AMP, cochl amp	heaping spoonful *(cochleare amplum)*
COCHL MAG, cochl mag	tablespoonful *(cochleare magnum)*

COCHL PARV, cochl parv	teaspoonful *(cochleare parvum)*
COCT, coct	boiling *(coctio)*
COL, col	strain *(cola)*
COLAT, colat	strained *(colatus)*
COLL, coll	eyewash *(collyrium)*
COLLUT, collut	mouthwash *(collutorium)*
COLLYR, collyr	eyewash *(collyrium)*
COMP	compound
CONT, cont	continue
CONT REM, cont rem	let the medicine be continued *(continuatur remedium)*
COQ, coq	boil *(coque)*
COQ IN S A, coq in s a	boil in sufficient water *(coque in sufficiente aqua)*
COQ S A, coq s a	boil properly *(coque secundum artem)*
CPD, cpd	compound
CUJ, cuj	of which *(cujus)*
CUJ LIB, cuj lib	of any you desire *(cujus libet)*
CV	tomorrow evening *(cras vespere)*
CVP lab	cardiovascular pulmonary laboratory
CW	clockwise

D	dose
	duration
	give *(da)*
	let it be given *(detur)*
	right *(dexter)*
d	day
DA, da	give *(da)*
dc, DC, D/C	discontinue
D/C	discharge
DD	let it be given to *(detur ad)*
DEB SPIS, deb spis	of the proper consistency *(debita spissitudo)*
DEC, dec	pour off *(decanta)*
DECR, decr	decrease
DECUB, decub	lying down *(decubitus)*
DE D IN D, de d in d	from day to day *(de die in diem)*
DEGLUT, deglut	let it be swallowed *(deglutiatur)*
DEST	distilled *(destillata)*
DET, det	let it be given *(detur)*
DIEB ALT, dieb alt	on alternate days *(diebus alternis)*
DIEB TERT, dieb tert	every third day *(diebus tertiis)*
DIG, dig	let it be digested *(digeratur)*
DIL, dil	dilute
DILUC, diluc	at daybreak *(diluculo)*

DILUT	dilute
D IN P AEQ, **d in p aeq**	divide into equal parts *(divide in partes* *aequales)*
DIR PROP, **dir prop**	with proper direction
DISC	discontinue
disch	discharge
DISP, disp	dispense
DIST, dist	distilled, distill
DIV, div	divide
DONEC ALV **SOL FUERIT,** **donec alv** **sol fuerit**	until the bowels are open *(donec alvus soluta fuerit)*
DP	with proper direction
DRSG	dressing
DTD	dispense of such a dose *(datur talis dosis)*
DTD No. vi	let six such doses be given
DTV	due to void
DUR DOLOR, **dur dolor**	while the pain lasts *(durante* *dolore)*
DW	distilled water
EAD, ead	the same *(eadem)*
EDC	estimated date of confinement expected date of confinement

EMP	as directed *(ex modo prescripto)*
EMUL	emulsion
ET, et	and
EVAL, eval	evaluation
EXHIB, exhib	let it be given *(exhibeatur)*
EXT, ext	extract
F	let it be made *(fiat)*
FEB DUR, feb dur	while the fever lasts *(febre durante)*
FERV, ferv	hot *(fervens)*
FF	fat free force fluids
FH, fh	let a draught be made *(fiat haustus)*
FILT, filt	filter
FL, fl	filtered load fluid
FLA, fla	according to rule *(fiat lege artis)*
FLD	fluid
FM	make a mixture *(fiat mistura)*
FP, fp	flat plate let a potion be made *(fiat potio)*
F PIL, f pil	let pills be made *(fiant pilulae)*

FRACT DOS, **fract dos**	in divided doses *(fracta dosi)*
freq	frequent
FSA, fsa	let it be made skillfully *(fiat secundum artem)*
FT, ft	let it be made *(fiat)*
FT MAS DIV IN PIL, **ft mas div in pil**	make a mass and divide into pills *(fiat massa dividenda in pilulae)*
FT PULV, ft pulv	make a powder *(fiat pulvis)*
F VS, f vs	let the patient be bled *(fiat venaesectio)*
GARG	gargle
GRAD	gradually, by degrees
H	hypodermic
HD, Hd	at bedtime *(hora decubitus)*
HEBDOM, hebdom	a week *(hebdomada)*
HOB	head of bed
HOR DECUB, **hor decub**	at bedtime *(hora decubitus)*
HOR INTERM **hor interm**	at intermediate hours *(horis intermediis)*
HOR SOM, hor som	at bedtime *(hora somni)*
HOR UN **SPATIO,** **hor un spatio**	at the end of an hour *(horae unius spatio)*

HS, hs	at bedtime *(hora somni)*
ID, id	the same *(idem)*
INCR, Incr	increase
IN D, in d	daily *(in die)*
INF, inf	pour in *(infunde)*
INJ ENEM, inj enem	let an enema be injected *(injiciatur enema)*
KVO	keep vein open
L	left
LIQ	liquid liquor
LOC DOL, loc dol	to the painful spot *(loco dolenti)*
lot	lotion
LT, lt	left
M	macerate mix
mac	macerate
MAN PR, man pr	early in the morning *(mane primo)*
MATUT, matut	in the morning *(matutinus)*
MB, mb	mix well *(misce bene)*
M DICT, m dict	as directed *(more dicto)*
M ET SIG, m et sig	mix and label *(misce et signa)*
M FT, m ft	make a mixture *(mistura fiat)*
MIST, mist	mixture *(mistura)*

MIT, mit	send *(mitte)*
MOD PRAESC, mod praesc	as directed *(modo prescripto)*
MOR DICT, mor dict	as directed *(more dicto)*
MOR SOL, mor sol	in the usual way *(more solito)*
MP, mp	as directed *(modo prescripto)*
M&R	measure and record
NB	note well *(nota bene)*
NBM	nothing by mouth
NOC, noc	night
NOCT, noct	at night *(nocte)*
NON REP, non rep	do not repeat *(non repetatur)*
NON REPETAT, non repetat	do not repeat *(non repetatur)*
NOS	not otherwise specified
NPO	nothing by mouth *(nulla per os)*
NPO/HS	nothing by mouth at bedtime *(nulla per os hora somni)*
NR	do not repeat *(non repetatur)*
Occ	occasional
OD	once daily
OJ, oj	orange juice

OM, om	every morning *(omni mane)*
OMN BIH, omn bih	every two hours *(omni bihora)*
OMN HOR, omn hor	every hour *(omni hora)*
OMN NOCT, omn noct	every night *(omni nocte)*
OM QUAR HOR, om quar hor	every quarter of an hour *(omni quarta hora)*
ON, on	every night *(omni nocte)*
OOB	out of bed
OTC	over the counter
P	after *(post)* position
P AE, p ae	in equal parts *(partes aequales)*
PAR AFF, par aff	the part affected *(pars affecta)*
PART AEQ, part aeq	in equal parts *(partes aequales)*
PART VIC, part vic	in divided doses *(partitis vicibus)*
PC, p.c.	after meals *(post cibum)*
per	by for each through
PER OS, per os	by mouth
PHAR	pharmacy
PHARM	pharmacy

PN	percussion note
PO	postoperative
PO, po	by mouth *(per os)*
POD	postoperative day
POT, pot	potion
PP	postpartum postprandial
PPA, ppa	shake well *(phiala prius agitata)*
PPT	precipitate
pr	through the rectum *(per rectum)*
PR	through the rectum *(per rectum)* prism
P RAT AETAT, p rat aetat	in proportion to age *(pro ratione aetatis)*
PRN, prn	as the occasion arises *(pro re nata)*
PTA, pta	prior to admission
PULM, pulm	gruel *(pulmentum)*
PULV, pulv	powder *(pulvis)*
pwd	powder
Q, q	each, every *(quaque)*
QAM, qam	every morning
QD, qd	every day *(quaque die)*
QH, qh	every hour *(quaque hora)*
q2h, q3h, q4h	every two hours, every three hours, every four hours

QHS, qhs	every bedtime
QID, qid	four times a day *(quater in die)*
QL, ql	as much as desired *(quantum libet)*
QM, qm	every morning *(quaque mane)*
QN, qn	every night *(quaque nocte)*
QNS, qns	quantity not sufficient
QOD, qod	every other day
QOH, qoh	every other hour
QP, qp	at will *(quantum placeat)*
QQH, qqh	every four hours *(quaque quarta hora)*
QQHOR, qqhor	every hour *(quaque hora)*
qs ad	to a sufficient quantity
QS, qs	enough *(quantum satis)* prepare sufficient volume
QSUFF, qsuff	as much as suffices *(quantum sufficit)*
QUOTID, quotid	daily *(quotidie)*
QV, qv	as much as you like *(quantum vis)*
R	right rub take *(recipe)*
RED IN PULV, red in pulv	reduced to powder *(reductus in pulverem)*

REP	let it be repeated *(repetatur)*
RO, R/O	rule out
ROM	range of motion
ROS	review of systems
Rot	rotate
RT	right
RX, Rx	prescription take *(recipe)* treatment
s, s̄	without *(sine)*
S	label *(signa)* left *(sinister)* sign *(signa)* without *(sine)* write *(signa)*
SAT, sat	saturated
SEQ LUCE, seq luce	the next day *(sequenti luce)*
serv	keep, preserve *(serva)*
Sig, sig	let it be labeled *(signetur)*
SIG N PRO, sig n pro	label with the proper name *(signa nomine proprio)*
SIMUL, simul	at the same time
SING, sing	of each *(singulorum)*
SI NON VAL, si non val	if it is not enough *(si non valeat)*
SI OP SIT, si op sit	if it is necessary *(si opus sit)*

SOL, sol	solution
SOLV, solv	dissolve *(solve)*
S OP SIT, s op sit	if it is necessary *(si opus sit)*
SOS	if it is necessary *(si opus sit)*, when necessary
S/P	status post
SPEC, spec	specimen
SS	soapsuds
SSS	layer upon layer *(stratum super stratum)*
SSV, ssv	under a poison label *(sub signo veneni)*
ST, st	let it stand *(stet)*
STAT, stat	immediately *(statim)*
std	standard
STET, stet	let it stand
SU, su	let him take *(sumat)*
SUM, sum	let him take *(sumat)*
SUM TAL, sum tal	let him take one like this *(sumat talem)*
SV, sv	alcoholic spirit *(spiritus vini)*
SVR, svr	rectified spirit of wine *(spiritus vini rectificatus)*
SVT, svt	proof spirit *(spiritus vini tenuis)*
SYR, syr	syrup
Tab	tablet
TAL, tal	of such, like this, such a one *(talis)*

T&C, T&X	test and crossmatch
TDS, tds	take three times a day *(ter die sumendum)*
TID, tid	three times a day *(ter in die)*
TKO	to keep open
TLC	tender loving care
TO	telephone order
TRIT, trit	triturate
UNG, ung	ointment *(unguentum)*
UNK	unknown
UTD	up to date
UT DICT, ut dict	as directed *(ut dictum)*
VIN, vin	wine *(vinum)*
VIZ	namely *(videlicet)*
VO, vo, V/O	verbal order
VOS, vos	dissolved in yolk of egg *(vitello ovi solutus)*
WNL	within normal limits
X-match	crossmatch

medical chemistry

A	acetum
	atropine
AA	acetic acid
	adenylic acid
	aggregated albumin
	aminoacetone
	amino acid
	Australia antigen
AAA	amalgam
	androgenic anabolic agent
AAAE	amino acid-activating enzymes
AAF	acetylaminofluorene
AAME	acetylarginine methyl ester
AAN	alpha-amino nitrogen
AAT	alpha-antitrypsin
AB	alcian blue
AC	anticoagulant
	anti-inflammatory corticoid
AcCoA	acetyl-coenzyme A
ACD	citric acid, trisodium citrate, dextrose (solution)
ACE	adrenocortical extract
	alcohol, chloroform, ether

119

acet.	acetone
	vinegar
AcG, Ac-G	accelerator globulin
ACH	adrenal cortical hormone
	acetylcholine
ACh, Ach	acetylcholine
AChE	acetylcholinesterase
ACI	aspiryl chloride
Acid PO$_4$	acid phosphatase
ACM	albumin, calcium, magnesium
ACP	acid phosphatase
	acyl-carrier protein
	aspirin, caffeine, phenacetin
ACPP	adrenocorticopolypeptide
ACS	antireticular cytotoxic serum
ACTH	adrenocorticotropic hormone
ACTP	adrenocorticotropin
	polypeptide
Acyl-Co A	organic compound-coenzyme
	A ester
ADA	adenosine deaminase
ADH	alcohol dehydrogenase
	antidiuretic hormone
ADP	adenosine diphosphate
ADPase	adenosine diphosphatase
Adr, adr	adrenaline
ADS	antidiuretic substance
ADT	adenosine triphosphate
AE	apoenzyme

AF	aldehyde fuchsin
A-F	antifibrinogen
AG	antiglobulin
AGL	aminoglutethimide
AGLMe	*N*-alpha-acetylglycyl-L-lysine methyl ester
AgNO₃	silver nitrate
AGV	aniline gentian violet
AH	acetohexamide aminohippurate antihyaluronidase
AHB	alpha-hydroxybutyric dehydrogenase
AHF	antihemolytic factor antihemophilic factor
AHG	antihemophilic globulin antihuman globulin
AHH	alpha-hydrazine analogue of histidine arylhydrocarbon hydroxylase
AHLS	antihuman-lymphocyte serum
AIA	allylisopropylacetamide
AIB	aminoisobutyric acid
AIC	aminoimidazole carboxamide
AIS	anti-insulin serum
AL	albumin
ALA	aminolevulinic acid
Alα	alanine
ALAD	aminolevulinic acid dehydrase

ALAS	aminolevulinic acid synthetase
ALB, Alb	albumin
alc	alcohol
ALD	aldolase
ALG	Annapolis lymphoblast globulin
	antilymphocyte globulin
ALH	anterior lobe hormone
Alk	alkaline
Alk PO$_4$	alkaline phosphatase
alk p'tase	alkaline phosphatase
ALME, ALMe	acetyl-L-lysine methyl ester
ALP	alkaline phosphatase
	antilymphocyte plasma
α-KG	alpha-ketoglutarate
α LP	alpha-lipoprotein
α_2M	alpha$_2$-macroglobulin
ALS	angiotensin-like substance
	antilymphatic serum
	antilymphocytic serum
ALTEE	acetyl-L-tyrosine ethyl ester
AM	alveolar macrophage
AMB	amphotericin B
AMD	alpha-methyldopa
AMG	antimacrophage globulin
AMI	amitriptyline
AMLS	antimouse-lymphocyte serum
AMM	ammonia

AMP	acid mucopolysaccharide
	adenosine monophosphate
	adenylic acid
	ampicillin
AMPS	acid mucopolysaccharides
AMP-S	adenylosuccinic acid
AMS	antimacrophage serum
AMT	alpha-methyltyrosine
	amethopterin
AMY	amylase
ANA	acetylneuraminic acid
	antinuclear antibodies
	aspartyl naphthylamide
ANF	alpha-naphthoflavone
	antinuclear factor
ANS	antineutrophilic serum
anti-HAA	antibody hepatitis-associated antigen
anti-S	anti-sulfanilic acid
AOAA	amino-oxyacetic acid
AP	acid phosphatase
	alkaline phosphatase
	aminopeptidase
APA	aminopenicillanic acid
	antipernicious anemia factor
APC	aspirin, phenacetin, caffeine
APC-C	aspirin, phenacetin, caffeine; with codeine
APE	aminophylline, phenobarbital, ephedrine
	anterior pituitary extract

APF	animal protein factor
APH	anterior pituitary hormone
APHP	antipseudomonas human plasma
APP	alum-precipitated pyridine
A-PRT	adenine phosphoribosyltransferase
APT	alum-precipitated toxoid
Arg	arginine
ARS	antirabies serum
AS	acetylstrophanthidin androsterone sulfate antistreptolysin
ASA	acetylsalicylic acid (aspirin) arylsulfatase-A
ASC	ascorbic acid
ASF	aniline, sulfur, formaldehyde
ASK	antistreptokinase
ASL	antistreptolysin
ASLO	antistreptolysin-O
ASN	alkali-soluble nitrogen
ASO	antistreptolysin-O antistreptolysin-O titer
Asp	aspartic acid
ASTO	antistreptolysin-O
ASV	antisnake venom
AT	aminotriazole antitrypsin
A.T. 10	dihydrotachysterol
ATA	anti-Toxoplasma antibodies aurintricarboxylic acid

ATE	adipose tissue extract
ATEe, ATEE	acetyltyrosine ethyl ester
ATG	antithyroglobulin
ATP	adenosine triphosphate
ATPase	adenosine triphosphatase
ATS	antitetanic serum antithymocyte serum
AU	azauridine
^{198}Au	radioactive gold
AUHAA	Australia hepatitis-associated antigen
AVP	8-arginine-vasopressin
AVT	8-arginine-oxytocin
AZG	azaguanine
AZUR	azauridine
BA	betamethasone acetate blocking antibody bovine albumin
Ba	barium
BAEE	benzoyl arginine ethyl ester benzylarginine ethyl ester
BAIB	beta-aminoisobutyric acid
BAL	British anti-lewisite (dimercaprol)
BAMe	benzoyl arginine methyl ester
BCB	brilliant cresyl blue
BCG	bacille Calmette-Guérin (vaccine)
BCP	birth control pill

BEI	butanol-extractable iodine (serum)
B-AIB, β**-AIB**	beta-aminoisobutyric acid
β **LP, BLP**	beta-lipoprotein
B/F	bound/free (antibody)
BGD	blood group-degrading (enzymes)
BGG	bovine gamma globulin
BGH	bovine growth hormone
BGP	beta-glycerophosphatase
BH	benzalkonium and heparin
BHA	butylated hydroxyanisole
BHC	benzene hexachloride
BHT	butylated hydroxytoluene
BIL, bil, bili	bilirubin
BIP	bismuth iodoform paraffin
BJP	Bence Jones protein
BLG	beta-lactoglobulin
BNG	6-bromo-2-naphthyl-beta-galactoside
BNGase	6-bromo-2-naphthyl-beta-galactosidase
B&O	belladonna and opium
BOEA	ethyl biscoumacetate
BP	benzopyrene
BPL	beta-propiolactone
BPO	benzylpenicilloyl
BR	bilirubin

BRM	biuret reactive material
BSA	bismuth-sulphite agar
	bovine serum albumin
BSI	bound serum iron
BSP	Bromsulphalein
	(sulfobromophthalein)
BSS	balanced salt solution
	buffered saline solution
BTSH,	beef thyroid-stimulating
B-TSH	hormone
	bovine thyroid-stimulating
	hormone
BUDR	bromodeoxyuracil
	bromodeoxyuridine
C	carbohydrate
	carbon
CA	catecholamine
	cytosine arabinoside
Ca	calcium
^{45}Ca	radioactive calcium
CaBP	calcium-binding protein
CaEDTA	calcium disodium edetate
	edathamil calcium disodium
cAMP	cyclic adenosine
	monophosphate
CAP	cellulose acetate phthalate
	chloramphenicol
	cystine aminopeptidase
CATH, cath	cathartic
CBG	corticosteroid-binding globulin
	cortisol-binding globulin

CC	compound cathartic
CCK	cholecystokinin
CCK-PZ	cholecystokinin pancreozymin
CDC	chenodeoxycholate
CDE	chlordiazepoxide
CDH	ceramide dihexoside
CDL	chlorodeoxylincomycin
CDP	cytidine diphosphate
CE	cholesterol esters
CEA	carcino-embryonic antigen
	crystalline egg albumin
CF	carbolfuchsin
	chemotactic factor
	Christmas factor
	citrovorum factor
Cf	iron *(ferrum)* carrier
CFA	complement-fixing antibody
	complete Freund adjuvant
Cf-Fe	carrier-bound iron
CG	cardio-green
	chorionic gonadotropin
	colloidal gold
	phosgene
CGP	choline glycerophosphatide
	chorionic growth hormone prolactin
CH	cholesterol
CHA	cyclohexylamine
CHE	cholinesterase
CHL	chloramphenicol

CHO	carbohydrate
CHOL, chol	cholesterol
CHOL E, chol est	cholesterol esters
CI	colloidal iron crystalline insulin
CK	creatine kinase
Cl	chloride chlorine
CLO	cod liver oil
CM	capreomycin carboxymethylcellulose chloroquine and mepacrine
CMB	carbolic methylene blue
CMC	carboxymethyl cellulose
CMP	cytidine monophosphate
CMT	catechol-O-methyl transferase
CN	cyanogen
CNL	cardiolipin natural lecithin
CNS	sulfocyanate
CO	carbon monoxide castor oil coenzyme
CO$_2$	carbon dioxide
COA, CoA	coenzyme A
COC	combination-type oral contraceptive
COHB, COHb	carboxyhemoglobin
COMT	catechol-O-methyl transferase

CP	chloropurine
	chloroquine and primiquine
	clottable protein
	coproporphyrin
	creatine phosphate
CPA	chlorophenylalanine
	cyclophosphamide
CPC	cetylpyridinium chloride
CPD	citrate, phosphate, dextrose
CPF	clot-promoting factor
CPIB	chlorophenoxyisobutyrate
CPK	creatine phosphokinase
CPP	cyclopentenophenanthrene
CPPD	calcium pyrophosphate dihydrate
CPS	chloroquine, pyrimethamine, sulfisoxazole
CPZ	chlorpromazine
CQ	chloroquine and quinine
CR	creatinine
	creatine phosphate
CRF	corticotropin-regulating (releasing) factor
Crit	hematocrit
CRM	cross-reacting material
CRP	C-reactive protein
CrP	creatine phosphate
	phosphocreatine
CS	chondroitin sulfate
	corticosteroid
	cycloserine

CSA	canavaninosuccinic acid
	chondroitin sulfate-A
CSF	colony-stimulating factor
CSL	cardiolipin synthetic lecithin
CT	chlorothiazide
CTAB	cetyltrimethylammonium bromide
CTC	chlortetracycline
CTFE	chlorotrifluoroethylene
CTH	ceramide trihexoside
CTP	cytidine triphosphate
CTP-^{3}H	cytidine triphosphate tritium-labeled
CTX	Cytoxan
CTZ	chlorothiazide
^{61}Cu, ^{64}Cu	radioactive copper
CV	cresyl violet
CY	cyanogen
CYCLO	cyclophosphamide
	cyclopropane
CZI	crystalline zinc insulin
D	deuterium
	deuteron
	dextrose
DA	dopamine
DAB	dimethylaminoazobenzene
DALA	delta-aminolevulinic acid
DAM	degraded amyloid
DAO	diamine oxidase

DAP	dihydroxyacetone phosphate
DAT	diphtheria antitoxin
DB	dextran blue
DBA	dibenzanthracene
DBI	phenethylbiguanide phenformin HCl
DBM	dibromomannitol
DC	deoxycholate diphenylarsine cyanide
DCA	deoxycholate-citrate agar desoxycorticosterone acetate
DCG	disodium cromoglycate
DCHFB	dichlorohexafluorobutane
DCI	dichloroisoproterenol
DCTMA	desoxycorticosterone trimethylacetate
DCTPA	desoxycorticosterone triphenylacetate
DDC	diethyldithiocarbamic acid dihydrocollidine
DDD	dichlorodiphenyldichloroethane
DDS	diaminodiphenylsulfone
DDT	dichlorodiphenyltrichloroethane
DEA	dehydroepiandrosterone
DEAE	diethylaminoethanol diethylaminoethyl
DEAE-D	diethylaminoethyl dextran
DEBA	diethylbarbituric acid
DEM	Demerol (meperidine)

DES	diethylstilbestrol
DET	diethyltryptamine
DEV	duck embryo vaccine
DF	desferrioxamine
DFDD	difluorodiphenyldichloroethane
DFDT	difluorodiphenyltrichloroethane
DFO	deferoxamine
DFP	diisopropylfluorophosphate
DFU	dideoxyfluorouridine
DG	deoxyglucose diglyceride
2DG	2-deoxy-D-glucose
DGVB	dextrose, gelatin, Veronal buffer
DHA	dehydroepiandrosterone dihydroxyacetone
DHAP	dihydroxyacetone phosphate
DHAS	dehydroepiandrosterone sulfate
DHE	dihydroergotamine
DHEA	dehydroepiandrosterone
DHEAS	dehydroepiandrosterone sulfate
DHFR	dihydrofolate reductase
DHIA	dehydroisoandrosterone
DHO	dihydroergocornine
DHT	dihydrotachysterol
DIP	diisopropyl phosphate
DIT	diiodotyrosine
DM	diphenylaminechlorarsine dopamine

DMA	dimethyladenosine
DMAB	dimethylaminobenzaldehyde
DMBA	dimethylbenzanthracene
DMCT	demethylchlortetracycline
DME	dimethyl ether (of *d*-tubocurarine)
DMM	dimethylmyleran
DMN	dimethylnitrosamine
DMO	dimethyloxazolidinedione
DMP	dimethylphthalate
DMPA	depomedroxyprogesterone acetate
DMPE	dimethoxyphenylethylamine
DMPEA	dimethoxyphenylethylamine
DMPP	dimethylphenylpiperazinium (iodide)
DMS, DMSO	dimethylsulfoxide
DMT	dimethyltryptamine
DNA	deoxyribonucleic acid
DNA-P	deoxyribonucleic acid phosphorus
DNase	deoxyribonuclease
DNB	dinitrobenzene
DNC	dinitrocarbanilide
DNCB	dinitrochlorobenzene
DNFB	dinitrofluorobenzene
DNOC	dinitro-*o*-cresol
DNP	deoxyribonucleoprotein dinitrophenol

DNPH	dinitrophenylhydrazine
DNPM	dinitrophenylmorphine
D5/N.S.	5 percent dextrose in normal saline
DO	diamine oxidase
DOC	deoxycholate deoxycorticosterone
DOCA	deoxycorticosterone acetate
DOCS	deoxycorticoids
DOET	dimethoxyethyl amphetamine
DOM	deaminated-O-methyl metabolite dimethoxymethyl amphetamine
DOMA	dihydroxymandelic acid
DON	diazo-oxonorleucine
DOPA, **Dopa**	dihydroxyphenylalanine
DOPAC	dihydroxyphenylacetic acid
DPA	diphenylamine dipropylacetate
DPD	desoxypyridoxine hydrochloride
DPG	diphosphoglycerate
DPGM	diphosphoglyceromutase
DPGP	diphosphoglycerate phosphatase
DPH	diphenylhydantoin (now phenytoin)
DPL	dipalmityl lecithin

DPN	diphosphopyridine nucleotide
	  (now nicotinamide adenine
	  dinucleotide)

DPNase	DPN hydrolyzing enzyme

DPNH	diphosphopyridine nucleotide, reduced (now nicotinamide adenine dinucleotide, reduced)
DPO	dimethoxyphenyl penicillin
DPS	demethylpolysiloxane
DPT	diphtheria toxoid, pertussis vaccine, tetanus toxoid dipropyltryptamine
DPTA	diethylenetriamine penta-acetic acid
DS	dehydroepiandrosterone sulfate dextrose-saline
D/S	dextrose in saline
DSC, DSCG	disodium cromoglycate
DSM	dextrose solution mixture
DTBC	*d*-tubocurarine
DTBN	di-*t*-butyl nitroxide
DTC	*d*-tubocurarine
DTMP	deoxythymidine monophosphate
DTNA	dithiobisnitrobenzoic acid
DTNB	dithiobisnitrobenzoic acid
DTPA	diethylenetriamine penta-acetic acid
DTT	dithiothreitol
DTZ	diatrizoate
DU	deoxyuridine

DUMP	deoxyuridine monophosphate
D/W	dextrose in water
D5/W, D-5-W, D-5/W, D_5W	5 percent dextrose in water
DX	dextran
DXM	dexamethasone
E	cortisone (compound E) epinephrine
E_1	estrone
E_2	estradiol
E_3	estriol
EA	ethacrynic acid
EACA	epsilon-aminocaproic acid
EAHLG	equine antihuman-lymphoblast globulin
EAHLS	equine antihuman-lymphoblast serum
EAP	epiallopregnanolone
EB	estradiol benzoate
EBI	emetine bismuth iodide
ECA	ethacrynic acid
ECP	erythrocyte coproporphyrin
EDTA	edathamil edetic acid ethylenediamine tetra-acetic acid
EEME	ethinylestradiol methyl ether
EFA	essential fatty acids

EGOT	erythrocyte glutamic oxaloacetic transaminase
EGS	ethylene glycol succinate
EHDP	ethane hydroxydiphosphate
EHF	exophthalmos-hyperthyroid factor
EI	enzyme inhibitor
EK	erythrokinase
EL, El, elix	elixir
EMB	eosin methylene blue ethambutol ethambutol-myambutol
EMF	erythrocyte maturation factor
ENA	extractable nuclear antigen
EO	ethylene oxide
EP	erythrocyte protoporphyrin
EPE	erythropoietin-producing enzyme
EPF	exophthalmos-producing factor
EPI	epinephrine
EPS	exophthalmos-producing substance
ESF	erythropoietic-stimulating factor
ESS	erythrocyte-sensitizing substance
ET	ethyl
ETA	ethionamide
ETH	elixir terpin hydrate
ETH/C	elixir terpin hydrate with codeine

ETM	erythromycin
ETOH, EtoH	ethyl alcohol
ETOX	ethylene oxide
ETT	extrathyroidal thyroxine
EWL	egg-white lysozyme
F	hydrocortisone (compound F)
FNα	filtered sodium
Fp	filtered phosphate
FA	fatty acid
	fluorescent antibody
	folic acid
	free acid
FAD	flavine adenine dinucleotide
FAN	fuchsin, amido black, and naphthol yellow
FBP	fibrinogen breakdown products
FBS	fetal bovine serum
FCA	ferritin-conjugated antibodies
FDP	fibrin degradation product
	fructose diphosphate
FDPase	fructose diphosphatase
Fe	iron
FEC, FECP	free erythrocyte coproporphyrin
FEP, FEPP	free erythrocyte protoporphyrin
FF	fixing fluid
FFA	free fatty acids
FFP	fresh frozen plasma
FG	fibrinogen

FGAR	formylglycinamide ribonucleotide
FI	fibrinogen
FIGLU	formiminoglutamic acid
FIT, FITC	fluorescein isothiocyanate
FM, FMN	flavin mononucleotide
FMS	fat-mobilizing substance
FP	frozen plasma
FPA	fluorophenylalanine
FPC	fish protein concentrate
FRC	frozen red cells
FRS	furosemide
FSF	fibrin-stabilizing factor
FSH	follicle-stimulating hormone
FSHRF	FSH-releasing factor
FSP	fibrinogen-split products
FT	free thyroxine
FTA	fluorescent treponemal antibody
FU	fecal urobilinogen fluorouracil
5-FU, 5-fu, 5FU	5-fluorouracil
FUDR	fluorodeoxyuridine
FUR	fluorouracil riboside
G	glucose immunoglobulin G
GA	glucuronic acid
GABA	gamma-aminobutyric acid

GAD	glutamic acid decarboxylase
γ-HCD	gamma-heavy chain disease protein
GAPD	glyceraldehyde phosphate dehydrogenase
GBA	ganglionic-blocking agent
GBH	graphite, benzalkonium, heparin
GC	glucocorticoid guanine cytosine
GDA	germine diacetate
GDH	glutamic dehydrogenase glycerophosphate dehydrogenase
GEE	glycine ethyl ester
GG	gamma globulin
GGG	gamboge
GGTP	gamma-glutamyl transpeptidase
GH	growth hormone
GHRF	growth hormone-releasing factor
GI	globin insulin
GIK	glucose, insulin, potassium
GIM	gonadotropin-inhibitory material
GIT	glutathione-insulin transhydrogenase
GK	glycerol kinase
GLOB, glob	globulin

GLU, glu	glucose
	glutamic acid
gly	glycerol
	glycine
GMA	glyceryl methacrylate
GMP	guanine monophosphate
	guanylic acid
G-MP	G-myeloma proteins
GOE	gas, oxygen, ether
GOT	glutamic oxaloacetic transaminase
GP	glutathione peroxidase
	glycoprotein
G-1-P	glucose-1-phosphate
GPAIS	guinea pig anti-insulin serum
GPC	glycerylphosphorylcholine
GPD	glucose phosphate dehydrogenase
G6PD	glucose-6-phosphate dehydrogenase
GPE	glycerylphosphorylethanolamine
GPI	glucosephosphate isomerase
GPK	guinea pig kidney (antigen)
GPS	guinea pig serum
GPT	glutamic pyruvic transaminase
GPUT	galactose phosphate uridyl transferase
GR	glutathione reductase
GRA	gonadotropin-releasing agent

GRF	gonadotropin-releasing factor
G/S	glucose and saline
GSA	guanidinosuccinic acid
GSH	glomerular-stimulating hormone reduced glutathione
GSSG	oxidized glutathione
GT	glutamyl transpeptidase
GTH	gonadotropic hormone
GTN	glyceryl trinitrate
GTP	glutamyl transpeptidase guanosine triphosphate
GV	gentian violet
H	hormone hydrogen
H antigens	flagella antigens
HA	hemagglutinating antibody hydroxyapatite
HAA	hepatitis-associated antigen
HABA	hydroxybenzeneazobenzoic acid
HAHTG	horse antihuman-thymus globulin
HAI	hemagglutination inhibition
HAL	halothane
HAP	histamine phosphate acid
HAPA	hemagglutinating antipenicillin antibody
HB, Hb	hemoglobin

Hb A	normal adult hemoglobin
Hb A$_2$	minor fraction of adult hemoglobin
HBABA	hydroxybenzeneazobenzoic acid
HBB	hydroxybenzyl benzimidazole
HBD, HBDH	hydroxybutyrate dehydrogenase
Hb F	fetal hemoglobin
HBI	high serum-bound iron
Hb M	hemoglobin M
HBO	hyperbaric oxygen
HbO$_2$	oxyhemoglobin
Hb S	sickle cell hemoglobin
HC	hepatic catalase hydroxycorticoid
HCC	hydroxycholecalciferol
HCG	human chorionic gonadotropin
HCH	hexachlorocyclohexane
HCl	hydrochloric acid
HCO$_3$	bicarbonate
HCP	hepatocatalase peroxidase
HCS	human chorionic somatomammotropin
17-HCS	17-hydroxycorticosteroids
HCSM	human chorionic somatomammotropin

HCT	hematocrit
	human chorionic placental thyrotropin
	hydrochlorothiazide
Hct	hematocrit
Hctz	hydrochlorothiazide
HDBH	hydroxybutyric dehydrogenase
HDC	histidine decarboxylase
HDL, HDLP	high-density lipoprotein
HDP	hydroxydimethylpyrimidine
He	helium
H&E	hematoxylin and eosin (stain)
HEC	hydroxyergocalciferol
HES	hydroxyethyl starch
HETP	hexaethyltetraphosphate
HF	Hageman factor
HFP	hexafluoropropylene
HFSH	human follicle-stimulating hormone
HG	hemoglobin
Hg	mercury
HGB, Hgb	hemoglobin
HGF	hyperglycemic-glycogenolytic factor
HGG	human gamma globulin
HGH	human growth hormone
HGPRT	hypoxanthine guanine phosphoribosyltransferase
HH	hydroxyhexamide

H&H	hemoglobin and hematocrit
HHB	un-ionized hemoglobin
HI	hydroxyindole
HIA	hemagglutination-inhibition antibody
5-HIAA	5-hydroxyindoleacetic acid
HIOMT	hydroxyindole-O-methyl transferase
His	histidine
HK	hexokinase
HL-A, HLA	human leukocyte antigen, a histocompatibility antigen
HLDH	heat-stable lactic dehydrogenase
HLH	human luteinizing hormone
HMF	hydroxymethylfurfural
HMG	human menopausal gonadotropin hydroxymethylglutaryl
HML	human milk lysozyme
HMM	hexamethylolmelamine
HMP	hexose monophosphate
HMPG	hydroxymethoxyphenylglycol
HMT	hematocrit
HN$_2$	nitrogen mustard, mechlorethamine
HNB	hydroxynitrobenzylbromide
HO	hyperbaric oxygen
HOC	hydroxycorticoid

HP, Hp	haptoglobin
HPAA	hydroxyphenylacetic acid
HPFSH	human pituitary follicle-stimulating hormone
HPG	human pituitary gonadotropin
HPL	human placental lactogen
HPLA	hydroxyphenyllactic acid
HPP	hydroxypyrazolopyrimidine
HPPA	hydroxyphenylpyruvic acid
HPPH	hydroxyphenyl-phenylhydantoin
HPS	hematoxylin, phloxine, saffron
HPV	*Hemophilus pertussis* vaccine
Hr	blood type factor
HRIG	human rabies immune globulin
HS	heme synthetase horse serum
HSA	human serum albumin
HS-Co A	reduced coenzyme A
3-HT	hydroxytyramine
5-HT	serotonin
HTA	hydroxytryptamine
HTOH	hydroxytryptophol
HTP	hydroxytryptophan
H-TSH	human thyroid-stimulating hormone
HUTHAS	human thymus antiserum
HVA	homovanillic acid
I	iodine

^{131}I, I$_{131}$	radioactive iodine
ICD	interstitial cell-stimulating hormone isocitric dehydrogenase
ICDH	isocitric dehydrogenase
ICG	indocyanine green
ICSH	interstitial cell-stimulating hormone
IDH	isocitric dehydrogenase
IDP	inosine diphosphate
IDU	idoxuridine iododeoxyuridine
IF	intrinsic factor
IFA	indirect fluorescent antibody
IG	immune globulin
Ig	immunoglobulin
IgA	immunoglobulin A
IgD	immunoglobulin D
IgE	immunoglobulin E
IgG	immunoglobulin G
IGH	idiopathic growth hormone
IgM	immunoglobulin M
IGP	intestinal glycoprotein
IHSA	iodinated human serum albumin
ileu	isoleucine
IMAA	iodinated macroaggregated albumin
IMP	inosine monophosphate inosinic acid
INAH	isonicotinic acid hydrazide

INH	isoniazid
	isoniazide
	isonicotinic acid hydrazide
IPC	isopropyl chlorophenyl
IPV	inactivated polio vaccine
IRG	immunoreactive glucagon
IRHCS	immunoradioassayable human chorionic somatomammotropin
IRHGH	immunoreactive human growth hormone
IRI	immunoreactive insulin
ISD, ISDN	isosorbide dinitrate
ISG	immune serum globulin
ISO	isoproterenol
ITP	inosine triphosphate
IUDR	iododeoxyuridine
K	potassium
KCl	potassium chloride
KFAB	kidney-fixing antibody
αKG	alpha-ketoglutarate
KGS	ketogenic steroid
KI	potassium iodide
KIA	Kligler iron agar
KLH	keyhole-limpet hemocyanin
KM	kanamycin
KMV	killed measles-virus vaccine
KPTI	Kunitz pancreatic trypsin inhibitor
KRB	Krebs-Ringer bicarbonate buffer

KRP	Krebs-Ringer phosphate
KRPS	Krebs-Ringer phosphate buffer solution
KS	ketosteroid
KV	killed vaccine
LA	lactic acid leucine aminopeptidase
LAA	leukocyte ascorbic acid
LAD	lactic acid dehydrogenase
LAH	lactalbumin hydrolysate
LAP	leucine aminopeptidase leukocyte alkaline phosphatase
LAS	linear alkylate sulfonate
LATS	long-acting thyroid stimulator
LBF	*Lactobacillus bulgaricus* factor
LBI	low serum-bound iron
LC	lipid cytosomes long-chain (triglycerides)
LCFA	long-chain fatty acids
LCL	Levinthal-Coles-Lillie cytoplasmic inclusion bodies
LCMG	long-chain monoglyceride
LCT	long-chain triglyceride
LD	lactic dehydrogenase L-dopa
LDH	lactate dehydrogenase lactic dehydrogenase
LDL, LDLP	low-density lipoprotein

L-dopa	L-dihydroxyphenylalanine levodopa
leu	leucine
LFN	lactoferrin
LH	luteinizing hormone
LHRF	luteinizing hormone-releasing factor
LL	lysolecithin
LLF	Laki-Lorand factor (fibrin- stabilizing factor, factor XIII)
LMD	low molecular weight dextran
LMDX	low molecular weight dextran
LMWD	low molecular weight dextran
LNPF	lymph node permeability factor
LP	lipoprotein lymphoid plasma
LPF	leukocytosis-promoting factor
LPL	lipoprotein lipase
LPS	lipopolysaccharide
LR	lactated Ringer's solution
LRF	liver residue factor luteinizing hormone-releasing factor
LRH	luteinizing hormone-releasing hormone
LRS	lactated Ringer's solution
LSD, LSD-25	lysergic acid diethylamide
LT	levothyroxine lymphotoxin

LTF	lipotrophic factor or hormone
LTH	lactogenic hormone luteotropic hormone
LTPP	lipothiamide pyrophosphate
LV	live vaccine
LVP	lysine-vasopressin
Lys	lysine
LZM	lysozyme
MA	mandelic acid
MAA	macroaggregated albumin
MAFH	macroaggregated ferrous hydroxide
MAM	methylazomethanol
Man-6-P	mannose-6-phosphate
MAO	monoamine oxidase
MAOI	monoamine oxidase inhibitor
MAP	methylacetoxyprogesterone methylaminopurine
MB	methylene blue
MBA	methylbovine albumin
MBAS	methylene blue active substance
MBD	methylene blue dye
MBP	melitensis, bovine, porcine (antigen)
MBSA	methylated bovine serum albumin
MC	medium-chain (triglycerides) mineralocorticoid mitomycin-C
MCA	methylcholanthrene

MCFA	medium-chain fatty acid
MCH	mean corpuscular hemoglobin
MCP	mitotic-control protein
MCT	medium-chain triglyceride
MD	malic dehydrogenase
MDA	methylenedioxyamphetamine
MDH	malic dehydrogenase
ME	mercaptoethanol
Me	methyl
MEA	mercaptoethylamine
MEG	mercaptoethylguanidine
MEP	meperidine
MER	methanol-extruded residue
Met	methionine
MF	5-methyltetrahydrofolate
MFP	monofluorophosphate
MG	monoglyceride
	methyl glucoside
Mg	magnesium
MGGH	methylglyoxal guanylhydrazone
MGH	monoglyceride hydrolase
MgSO$_4$	magnesium sulfate
MH	mammotropic hormone
MHA	methemalbumin
MHb	methemoglobin
MHP	mercurihydroxypropane
MHPE	3-methoxy-4-hydroxyphenylethanol

MHPG	methoxyhydroxyphenylglycol
MI	mercaptoimidazole
MIF	macrophage-inhibiting factor
	migration-inhibition factor
MIT	monoiodotyrosine
MKV	killed measles vaccine
MMA	methylmalonic acid
MMPR	methylmercaptopurine riboside
MMR	measles, mumps, rubella
MO	mineral oil
MOM	milk of magnesia
MOMA	methoxyhydroxymandelic acid
MOPV	monovalent oral poliovirus vaccine
MP	mercaptopurine
	methylprednisolone
	monophosphate
	mucopolysaccharide
MPA	medroxyprogesterone acetate
	methylprednisolone acetate
MPC	marine protein concentrate
	meperidine, promethazine,
	chlorpromazine
MPEH	methylphenylethylhydantoin
MPO	myeloperoxidase
MPP	mercaptopyrazidopyrimidine
MPS	mucopolysaccharide
MR	methyl red
	muscle relaxant
MR-E	methemoglobin reductase

mRNA	messenger ribonucleic acid
MS	morphine sulfate
MSG	monosodium glutamate
MSH	melanocyte-stimulating hormone melanophore-stimulating hormone
MSLA	mouse-specific lymphocyte antigen
MSU	monosodium urate
MT	methoxytyramine methyltyrosine
MTHF	methyltetrahydrofolic acid
MTT	monotetrazolium
MTU	methylthiouracil
MTX	methotrexate
MUC	mucilage
MU-GAL	methylumbelliferyl- β-galactosidase
NA	neutralizing antibody noradrenalin
Na	sodium
NaCl	sodium chloride
NAD	nicotinamide adenine dinucleotide
NADH	nicotinamide adenine dinucleotide (reduced form)
NADP	nicotinamide adenine dinucleotide phosphate

NADPH	nicotinamide adenine dinucleotide phosphate (reduced form)
NANA	N-acetylneuraminic acid
NAPA	N-acetyl-p-aminophenol
NB	nitrous oxide-barbiturate
NBS	normal burro serum
NBT	nitroblue tetrazolium
NDGA	nordihydroguaiaretic acid
NDMA	nitrosodimethylaniline
NE	norepinephrine
NEFA	nonesterified fatty acids
NEM	N-ethylmaleimide
NGF	nerve growth factor
NHS	normal horse serum normal human serum
NM	normetadrenaline
Nm	nutmeg
NMN	nicotinamide mononucleotide normetanephrine
N₂O	nitrous oxide
NOR	noradrenaline
NP	normal plasma nucleoprotein
NPD	natriuretic plasma dialysate
NPH	neutral protamine Hagedorn (insulin)
NPN	nonprotein nitrogen

NRS	normal rabbit serum
	normal reference serum
NS	normal saline
N/S	normal saline
NSS	normal saline solution
NTA	nitrilotriacetic acid
NTAB	nephrotoxic antibody
NTG	nitroglycerin
O_2	oxygen
O_3	ozone
OA	oxalic acid
O&B	opium and belladonna
OC, OCP	oral contraceptive
OCT	ornithine carbamyltransferase
OF	Ovenstone factor
OGS	oxogenic steroid
OHC	hydroxycholecalciferol
OHCS, OHCs	hydroxycorticosteroids
OH-DOC	hydroxydeoxycorticosterone
OHFA	hydroxy fatty acid
OH IAA	hydroxyindoleacetic acid
OHP	oxygen under high pressure
OIH	orthoiodohippurate
Ol	oil
Ol res	oleoresin
OLH	ovine lactogenic hormone
OLP	abnormal lipoprotein

OMPA	octamethylpyrophosphoramide
ONP	ortho-nitrophenyl
ONPG	o-nitrophenyl-β-galactoside
ONP-GAL	ortho-nitrophenyl-β-galactosidase
OPG	oxypolygelatin
OPV	oral poliovirus vaccine
OT	old tuberculin
OTC	ornithine transcarbamylase oxytetracycline
OX, ox	oxymel
P	phosphorus protein
32p, P231	radioactive phosphorus
PAB, PABA	para-aminobenzoic acid
PAC	phenacetin, aspirin, codeine
PAH	para-aminohippurate para-aminohippuric acid polycyclic aromatic hydrocarbon
PAHA	para-aminohippuric acid
PAM	crystalline penicillin G in 2% aluminum monostearate phenylalanine mustard pralidoxime chloride pyridine aldoxime methiodide
PAN	peroxyacetyl nitrate
PANS	puromycin aminonucleoside
PAP	prostatic acid phosphatase
PAPP	para-aminopropiophenone

PAPS	phosphoadenosyl-phosphosulfate
PAS	para-aminosalicylic acid
PASA	para-aminosalicylic acid
PAS-C	para-aminosalicylic acid crystallized with ascorbic acid
PASM	periodic acid-silver methenamine
PB, Pb	phenobarbital
PBG	porphobilinogen
PB-Fe	protein-bound iron
PBI	protein-bound iodine
PBO	penicillin in beeswax placebo
PBS	phosphate-buffered saline phosphate-buffered sodium
PBT_4	protein-bound thyroxine
PBZ	pyribenzamine
PC	phosphocreatine phosphatidylcholine platelet concentrate pyruvate carboxylase
PCA	perchloric acid phenylcarboxylic acid
PCD	phosphate, citrate, dextrose
PCF	prothrombin conversion factor
p-CMB	parachloromercuribenzoate
PCN, pcn	penicillin
PCP	parachlorophenate
PCPA	parachlorophenylalanine

PD	phosphate dehydrogenase
	porphobilinogen deaminase
PDA	predialyzed human albumin
PDAB	paradimethylaminobenzaldehyde
PDG	phosphogluconate dehydrogenase
PDH	phosphate dehydrogenase
PDP	piperidino-pyrimidine
PDS	predialyzed human serum
PE	phenylephrine
	phosphatidylethanolamine
	polyethylene
PEBG	phenethylbiguanide
PEG	polyethylene glycol
pen	penicillin
PEP	phosphoenolpyruvate
PETN	pentaerythritol tetranitrate
PF	platelet factor
PFIB	perfluoroisobutylene
PFK	phosphofructokinase
PFU	plaque-forming units
PG	plasma triglyceride
	phosphogluconate
	prostaglandin
PGA	prostaglandin A
	pteroylglutamic acid
PGD	phosphogluconate dehydrogenase
	phosphoglyceraldehyde dehydrogenase
PGDH	phosphogluconate dehydrogenase

PGE	platelet granule extract prostaglandin E
PGF	prostaglandin F
PGH	pituitary growth hormone plasma growth hormone
PGI	phosphoglucoisomerase potassium, glucose, insulin
PGK	phosphoglycerate kinase
PGM	phosphoglucomutase
PH	phenyl
PHA	phenylalanine phytohemagglutinin
PHA-M	phytohemagglutinin M
PHBB	propylhydroxybenzyl benzimidazole
phe	phenylalanine
PHI	phosphohexoisomerase
PHK	platelet phosphohexokinase
PI	phosphatidylinositol proinsulin protamine insulin
PIF	prolactin-inhibiting factor
PII	plasma inorganic iodine
P-IRI	plasma immunoreactive insulin
pit	pitocin
PK	pyruvate kinase
PKA	prokininogenase
PKV	killed poliomyelitis vaccine

PL	phospholipid
	placebo
	placental lactogen
PLS	prostaglandin-like substance
PLV	live poliomyelitis vaccine
	phenylalanine, lysine, vasopressin
PMB	parahydroxymercuribenzoate
PMI	phosphomannose isomerase
PMS	phenazine methosulfate
	postmitochondrial supernatant
	pregnant mare serum
PMSG	pregnant mare serum gonadotropin
PNA	pentosenucleic acid
PNC	penicillin
PNP	paranitrophenol
PNPG	p-nitrophenyl-β-galactoside
PNPP	paranitrophenylphosphate
POB	phenoxybenzamine
pOH	hydroxyl concentration
POPOP	p-bis(2-(5-phenyloxazolyl)) benzene
POT	potion
PP	prothrombin-proconvertin
	protoporphyrin
	pyrophosphate
PPA	phenylpyruvic acid
PPCF	plasma prothrombin conversion factor

PPD	paraphenylenediamine purified protein derivative
PPF	pellagra preventive factor
PPH	protocollagen proline hydroxylase
PPL	protein-polysaccharide
PPO	diphenyloxazole
PQ	pyrimethamine-quinine
PR	protein
PRC	packed red cells
PRI	phosphoribose isomerase
PRM	phosphoribomutase
PRO	protein prothrombin
PRP	platelet-rich plasma polymer of ribose phosphate
PRPP	phosphoribosylpyrophosphate
PRT	phosphoribosyltransferase
PS	chloropicrin phosphatidylserine
PSA	polyethylene sulfonic acid
PSC	Porter-Silber chromogen
PSP	phenolsulfonphthalein
PSS	physiologic saline solution
PST	penicillin, streptomycin, tetracycline
PTA	phosphotungstic acid plasma thromboplastin antecedent
PTAH	phosphotungstic acid hematoxylin

PTC	phenylthiocarbamide
	plasma thromboplastin component
PTE	parathyroid extract
PTH	parathormone
	parathyroid hormone
PTMA	phenyltrimethylammonium
PTS	para-toluenesulfonic acid
PTU	propylthiouracil
PUFA	polyunsaturated fatty acid
PVA	polyvinyl alcohol
PVC	polyvinyl chloride
PVP	penicillin V potassium
	polyvinylpyrrolidone
PZ	pancreozymin
PZA	pyrazinamide
PZ-CCK	pancreozymin-cholecystokinin
PZI	protamine zinc insulin
QC	quinine and colchicine
Ra	radium
RADTS	rabbit antidog-thymus serum
RAI	radioactive iodine
RAMT	rabbit antimouse thymocyte
RARLS	rabbit antirat-lymphocyte serum
RATHAS	rat thymus antiserum
RBA	rose bengal antigen
RBP	retinol-binding protein
RCF	red cell folate

RDE	receptor-destroying enzyme
REF	renal erythropoietic factor
Rh	Rhesus blood factor
RI	radioisotope
RIFA	radioiodinated fatty acid
RIHSA	radioactive iodinated human serum albumin
RISA, risa	radioiodinated serum albumin
RITC	rhodamine isothiocyanate
RLS	Ringer's lactate solution
RNA	ribonucleic acid
RNase	ribonuclease
RNP	ribonucleoprotein
RP	reactive protein
R-5-P	ribose-5-phosphate
RPR	rapid plasma reagin
RPS	renal pressor substance
RR-HPO	rapid recompression-high pressure oxygen
RTF	resistance transfer factor
RVP	red veterinary petrolatum
SA	salicylic acid saline serum albumin
SAL	saline
SAM	sulfated acid mucopolysaccharide
SAP	serum alkaline phosphatase
SB	serum bilirubin

SBTI	soybean trypsin inhibitor
SC	succinylcholine
SCFA	short-chain fatty acid
SCH	succinylcholine
SCK	serum creatine kinase
SCOP	scopolamine
SCP	single-celled protein
SCPK, S-CPK	serum creatine phosphokinase
SD	streptodornase
SDH	serine dehydrase sorbitol dehydrogenase succinate dehydrogenase
SDS	sodium dodecyl sulfate
SG	serum globulin
SGOT	serum glutamic oxaloacetic transaminase
SGP	serine glycerophosphatide soluble glycoprotein
SGPT	serum glutamic pyruvic transaminase
SH	sex hormone somatotropic hormone sulfhydryl
SHB	sulfhemoglobin
SHBD	serum hydroxybutyrate dehydrogenase
SHG	synthetic human gastrin
SI	serum iron soluble insulin
SICD	serum isocitric dehydrogenase

SK	streptokinase
SK-SD	streptokinase-streptodornase
SL	streptolysin
SLAP	serum leucine aminopeptidase
SLD	serum lactic dehydrogenase
SLDH	serum lactic dehydrogenase
SLO	streptolysin-O
SM	streptomycin
SMP	slow-moving protease
SOC	sequential-type oral contraceptive
SOM	sulformethoxine
SOTT	synthetic medium old tuberculin trichloroacetic acid precipitated
SPBI	serum protein-bound iodine
SPCA	serum prothrombin-conversion accelerator
SPI	serum precipitable iodine
SRF	somatotropin-releasing factor
SRNA	soluble ribonucleic acid
SRS	slow-reacting substance
SSA	salicylsalicylic acid skin-sensitizing antibody
SSKI	saturated solution of potassium iodide
STA	serum thrombotic accelerator
STH	somatotropic hormone
STK	streptokinase
STM	streptomycin

STP	scientifically treated petroleum
SUA	serum uric acid
SUN	serum urea nitrogen
SV	snake venom
T_3	triiodothyronine
T_4	thyroxine, levothyroxine, tetraiodothyronine
TA	alkaline tuberculin titratable acid toxin-antitoxin
TA_4	tetraiodothyroacetic acid
TAB	typhoid, paratyphoid A, and paratyphoid B vaccine
TACE	tripara-anisylchloroethylene
TAF	albumose-free tuberculin toxoid-antitoxin floccules trypsin, aldehyde, fuchsin
TAM	toxin-antitoxin mixture
TAME, TAMe	toluenesulphotrypsin arginine methyl ester
TAO	triacetyloleandomycin
TAT	tetanus antitoxin toxin-antitoxin tyrosine aminotransferase
TB	toluidine blue
TBA	tertiary butylacetate thiobarbituric acid thyroxine-binding albumin
TBC	thyroxine-binding coagulin
TBG	thyroxine-binding globulin

TBN	bacillus emulsion
TBP	thyroxine-binding protein
TBPA	thyroxine-binding prealbumin
TBS	tribromosalicylanilide triethanolamine-buffered saline
TC	taurocholate tetracycline tubocurarine
TCA	tricarboxylic acid trichloroacetate trichloroacetic acid
TCAP	trimethylcetylammonium pentachlorophenate
TCC	trichlorocarbanilide
TCDC	taurochenodeoxycholate
TCE	trichloroethylene
TCP	therapeutic continuous penicillin
TCSA	tetrachlorosalicylanilide
TCT	thyrocalcitonin
TDC	taurodeoxycholate
TDI	toluene-diisocyanate
TDP	thymidine diphosphate
TEA	tetraethylammonium
TEAB	tetraethylammonium bromide
TEAC	tetraethylammonium chloride
TEB	tris-ethylenediaminetetra-acetate borate
TEE	tyrosine ethyl ester
TEEP	tetraethyl pyrophosphate

TEIB	triethyleneiminobenzoquinone
TEL	tetraethyl lead
TEM	triethylenemelamine
TEPA	triethylenephosphoramide
TEPP	tetraethyl pyrophosphate
TES	trismethylaminoethanesulfonic acid
TETD	tetraethylthiuram disulfide
TETRAC	tetraiodothyroacetic acid
TF	transfer factor tuberculin filtrate
Tf	transferrin
TFE	tetrafluoroethylene
Tf-Fe	transferrin-bound iron
TG	testosterone glucuronide thioguanine thyroglobulin triglyceride
TGFA	triglyceride fatty acid
TGL	triglyceride triglyceride lipase
THA	total hydroxyapatite
THAM	trihydroxymethylaminomethane
THC	tetrahydrocannabinol
THDOC	tetrahydrodeoxycorticosterone
THE	tetrahydrocortisone
THF	thymic humoral factor tetrahydrocortisol tetrahydrofolic acid

THFA	tetrahydrofolic acid
	tetrahydrofurfuryl alcohol
THI	trihydroxyindole
Thio-TEPA	triethylene thiophosphoramide
THO	tritiated water
THP	total hydroxyproline
tinct	tincture
TK	thymidine kinase
TMCA	trimethyl colchicinic acid
TMG	3,3-tetramethyleneglutaric acid
TML	tetramethyl lead
TMP	thymidine monophosphate
	trimethoprim
TMS	trimethylsilyl
TMTD	tetramethylthiuram disulfide
TNT	trinitrotoluene
TO	original tuberculin
	tincture of opium
TOCP	triorthocresyl phosphate
TOPV	trivalent oral poliovirus vaccine
TP	thymidine phosphorylase
	total protein
	tryptophan
	tube precipitin
TPI	triose phosphate isomerase
TPM	triphenylmethane
TPN	triphosphopyridine nucleotide

TPNH	reduced triphosphopyridine nucleotide
TPP	thiamine pyrophosphate
TPS	tumor polysaccharide substance
TPT	typhoid-paratyphoid (vaccine)
TPTZ	tripyridyltriazine
TR, tr	tincture
TR	tuberculin R (new tuberculin)
TRA	transaldolase
TRF	thyrotropin-releasing factor
TRH	thyrotropin-releasing hormone
Triac	triiodothyroacetic acid
Trig	triglycerides
TRIT	triiodothyronine
TRK	transketolase
TRMC	tetramethylrhodamino-isothiocyanate
TROCH	trochiscus
TSA	trypticase soy agar type-specific antibody
TSB	trypticase soy broth
TSC	thiosemicarbazide
TSE	trisodium edetate
TSF	tissue coding factor
TSH	thyroid-stimulating hormone
TSI	triple sugar iron (agar)
TSTA	tumor-specific transplantation antigen

TSY	trypticase soy yeast
TTC	triphenyltetrazolium chloride
TTH	thyrotropic hormone
TTP	thymidine triphosphate
TU	thiouracil
Tyr	tyrosine
TZ	tuberculin zymoplastiche
UA	uric acid
UCBR	unconjugated bilirubin
UCG	urinary chorionic gonadotropin
UCP	urinary coproporphyrin
UD	uroporphyrinogen decarboxylase
UDP	uridine diphosphate
UDPG	uridine diphosphoglucose
UDPGA	uridine diphosphoglucuronic acid
UDPgal	uridine diphosphate galactose
UDPGT	uridine diphosphoglucuronyl-transferase
UFA	unesterified fatty acids
UI	uroporphyrinogen isomerase
UIF	undegraded insulin factor
UK	urokinase
UM	uracil mustard
UMP	uridine monophosphate
UN	urea nitrogen
UP	uroporphyrin
UPG	uroporphyrinogen
URF	uterine-relaxing factor

UTBG	unbound thyroxine-binding globulin
UTP	uridine triphosphate
UU	urine urobilinogen
UUP	urine uroporphyrin
vac	vaccine
VAMP	vincristine, amethopterin, 6-mercaptopurine, prednisone
VB	vinblastine
VBS	Veronal-buffered saline
VBS:FBS	Veronal-buffered saline-fetal bovine serum
VC, VCR	vincristine
VDEM, VDM	vasodepressor material
VDP	vincristine, daunorubicin, prednisone
V&E	Vinethene and ether
VEM	vasoexcitor material
VHDL	very high-density lipoprotein
VIA	virus-inactivating agent
VIG	vaccinia immune globulin
Vin	vinyl ether
VIP	vasoactive intestinal peptide
VLDL	very low-density lipoprotein
VM, Vm	viomycin
VMA	vanillylmandelic acid
VP	vasopressin
VS	volumetric solution

VT	vacuum tuberculin
VV	viper venom
V-Z	varicella-zoster (antibody)
WRE	whole ragweed extract
Z/G, ZIG	zoster immune globulin

terms of measurement/ organisms

Measurement terms

A	absorbance
	age
	ampere
	angstrom
	annum
	area
	mass number
	total acidity
AA	achievement age
AAP	air at atmospheric pressure
AET, **aet**	age *(aetas)*
	aged *(aetatis)*
amp	ampere
	ampule
amp-hr	ampere-hour
AQ	achievement quotient
ATA	atmosphere absolute
AU	Angström unit
AV	avoirdupois

B	Baumé's scale
	Benoist's scale
BE	base excess
BEV, bev	billion electron volts
BP, bp	boiling point
BSU	British Standard Unit
BThU	British Thermal Unit
BTU	British Thermal Unit
BU	Bodansky unit
C	Celsius
	centigrade
	gallon
	hundred
	large (kilogram) calorie
	speed of light
c	curie
	small (gram) calorie
c'	coefficient of partage
CA	chronologic age
ca	about *(circa)*
Cal	large (kilogram) calorie
cal	small (gram) calorie
cc	cubic centimeter
CEL	Celsius
CENT	centigrade
cent	centimeter
centi-	hundred
CF	contractile force
cg	centigram

cgm	centigram
CGS	centimeter-gram-second (system)
Ci	curie
cl	centiliter
cm	centimeter
cm^3	cubic centimeter
c/min	cycles per minute
cmm	cubic millimeter
cong	gallon
CP	candle power constant pressure
cp	candle power centipoise
cpm	counts per minute cycles per minute
cps	cycles per second
CS	current strength
cu cm	cubic centimeter
cu ft	cubic foot
cu in	cubic inch
cu m	cubic meter
cu mm	cubic millimeter
cwt	hundredweight
D	density diopter
d	density diameter dyne
db	decibel

DC, dc	direct current
deca-	ten
decem	ten, a tenth
deci-	a tenth
DECR, decr	decrease(d) diminish(ed)
DEG	degree
dg	decigram
dgm	decigram
DIM, dim	one-half *(dimidius)*
dl	deciliter
dm	decimeter
dpm	disintegrations per minute
DQ	developmental quotient
dr	dram
DV, dv	double vibration
E	electromotive force
EF	ejection fraction
EMF, emf	electromotive force
EMU, emu	electromagnetic unit
Eq	equivalent(s)
ESE	electrostatic unit
ESU, esu	electrostatic unit
EU	Ehrlich unit
eV, ev	electron volt
F	Fahrenheit French (catheter size) gilbert (unit of magnetomotive force)

FAHR	Fahrenheit
FB, Fb	fingerbreadth
FF	filtration fraction
FFT	flicker fusion threshold
fl dr	fluid dram
fl oz	fluid ounce
FP	freezing point
fps	frames per second
FR, Fr	French (catheter size)
ft	foot
ft-c	foot-candle
ft-lb	foot-pound
FX	fractional
G	force (the pull of gravity)
	gram
g	gram
	gravity
g%	g/dl
	g/100 ml
	gram percent
ga	gauge
gal	gallon
g-cal	gram-calorie
g-cm	gram-centimeter
GL	greatest length
Gm, gm	gram
Gm%, gm%	grams per hundred milliliters
gm-m	gram-meter
GMW	gram-molecular weight

gr	grain(s)
gt	drop
gtt	drops
H	henry
	Holzknecht unit
	hour
h	hour
HED	unit of roentgen-ray dosage *(Haut-Einheits-Dosis)*
HPF, hpf	high power field
hr	hour
HT, ht, Hgt	height
HVL	half-value layer
I	intensity of magnetism
IA	impedance angle
ID	inside diameter
IE	immunizing unit
in	inch
IQ	intelligence quotient
IU	immunizing unit
	international unit
J	Joule's equivalent
K	absolute zero
	electrostatic capacity
	Kelvin
k	a constant
KA	King-Armstrong unit
kc	kilocycle
kcal	kilocalorie

kcps	kilocycles per second
kev	kiloelectron volt
kg	kilogram
kg-cal	kilogram-calorie
kg-m	kilogram-meter
KHZ	kilohertz
km	kilometer
kv	kilovolt
kva	kilovolt-ampere
kvcp	kilovolt constant potential
kvp	kilovolt peak
kw	kilowatt
kw-hr	kilowatt-hour
L	coefficient of induction
	length
	liter
	pound *(libra)*
l	liter
lb	pound *(libra)*
LF	limit of flocculation
LIB, lib	pound *(libra)*
LPF, lpf	low power field
lpm	liters per minute
M	handful *(manipulus)*
	minim
	molar
	thousand
m	meter
	minim

MA	mental age
ma, mA	milliampere
mam	milliampere minute
MAN, man	handful *(manipulus)*
mas	milliampere second
MAX, Max, max	maximum
MC	megacurie
	megacycle
mc	millicurie
mcg	microgram
mch	millicurie hour
mCi	millicurie
Mcps	megacycles per second
MCV	mean clinical value
MED	median
mEq, MEq, meq	milliequivalent
mEq/L	milliequivalents per liter
mev	million electron volts
Mf	microfilaria
mf	millifarad
M/F	male-female ratio
mg	milligram
mg%	milligrams percent
mg-el	milligram-element (radioactive)
mgh	milligram-hour (radioactivity)
mg-hr	milligram-hour (radioactivity)

mgm	milligram
mHg, mmHg	millimeters of mercury
MIN, min	minim
	minimal
	minimum
	minute
MKS	meter-kilogram-second
ml	milliliter
mm	millimeter
mM	millimols, millimoles
mM/L	millimols per liter
mmm	millimicron
mmole	millimol
mmpp	millimeters partial pressure
mN	millinormal
MOD, mod	moderate
MOL WT, mol wt	molecular weight
mOsm	milliosmol
MP, mp	melting point
mr	milliroentgen
mrad	millirad
mrem	millirem
msec	millisecond
mU	milliunit
mu	micron
mv, mV	millivolt
MW	molecular weight

my	mayer (unit of heat capacity)
NA	numeric aperture
nc	nanocurie
NEG, neg	negative
ng	nanogram (millimicrogram)
nl	nanoliter (millimicroliter) normal limits
nM	nanomolar (millimicromolar)
NR	normal range
O	pint *(octarius)*
OD	optical density outside diameter
oz	ounce
P	handful *(pugillus)* near point weight *(pondus)*
PC	weight *(pondus civile)*
pc	picocurie
PD	potential difference prism diopter
PE, Pe	probable error
pg	picogram
pH	hydrogen ion concentration, measure of alkalinity and acidity
PKV	peak kilovolts
pl	picoliter
POCUL, pocul	cup *(poculum)*

POS, pos	positive
PP	near point (*punctum proximum*)
PPB, ppb	parts per billion
PPM, ppm	parts per million
PQ	permeability quotient
PR	far point (*punctum remotum*)
	production rate
PS, ps	per second
psi	pounds per square inch
psia	pounds per square inch absolute
psig	pounds per square inch gauge
PT	pint
Q	coulomb
	electric quantity
	quart
QS, qs	enough (*quantum satis*)
qt	quart
QUAT, quat	four (*quattuor*)
QUINQ, quinq	five (*quinque*)
QUINT, quint	fifth (*quintus*)
R	Behnken's unit
	Rankine (scale)
	Réaumur (scale)
	resistance (electrical)
	roentgen
rad	radiation absorbed dose

RBE	relative biological effectiveness (of radiation)
rd	rutherford
REM	roentgen-equivalent—man
REP	roentgen-equivalent—physical
RH	relative humidity
rpm	revolutions per minute
S	half *(semis)* single Svedberg unit of sedimentation coefficient
SA	surface area
SCR, scr	scruple
SD	standard deviation
SE	standard error
SEE	standard error of the estimate
SEM	standard error of the mean
SEMID, semid	half a dram
SEMIH, semih	half an hour
SG, Sg	specific gravity
SP GR, sp gr	specific gravity
sq cm	square centimeter
sq m	square meter
sq mm	square millimeter
ss	one-half *(semis)*
SSD	source to skin distance sum of square deviations

stat	German unit of radium emanation
T, temp	temperature
T$\frac{1}{2}$	half-life
tbsp	tablespoonful
TRU	turbidity-reducing unit
tsp	teaspoonful
TU	toxic unit tuberculin unit
U	unit
UHF	ultra high frequency
v	volt volume
va	volt-ampere
VIB, vib	vibration
VOL, vol	volume
vs	vibration seconds
W	wehnelt (unit of hardness of roentgen rays)
w	watt
WL, wl	wavelength
WT, wt	weight
w/v	weight per volume
X	homeopathic symbol for the decimal scale of potencies Kienböck's unit of X-ray dosage
yd	yard
yr(s)	year(s)
z	atomic number

Organisms

A	*Actinomyces*
	Anopheles
AFB	acid-fast bacillus
B	bacillus
	Brucella
BACT, Bact	bacterium
BCG	bacille Calmette-Guérin
BHS	beta-hemolytic streptococci
BR	*Brucella*
BVV	bovine vaginitis virus
C	*Cimex*
	Clostridium
	Corynebacterium
	Cryptococcus
	Culex
CA	croup-associated virus
CEEV	Central European encephalitis virus
CHR	*Chromobacterium*
CL, cl	*Clostridium*
CMV	cytomegalovirus
E	*Entamoeba*
	Escherichia
EB, EBV	Epstein-Barr virus
EC	*Escherichia coli*
ECHO	enteric cytopathogenic human orphan virus
E coli	*Escherichia coli*

EEC, EPEC	enteropathogenic *Escherichia coli*
ESCH	*Escherichia*
F	*Filaria* *Fusobacterium*
FAV	feline ataxia virus
G	gonidial colony
GC, gc	gonococcus
GNID	gram-negative intracellular diplococci
H	Hauch (motile) *Hemophilus*
HKLM	heat-killed *Listeria monocytogenes*
HLV	herpes-like virus
HSV	herpes simplex virus
HTV	herpes-type virus
KL bac	Klebs-Löffler bacillus (diphtheria)
Kleb	*Klebsiella*
L	*Lactobacillus* *Leishmania*
LDV	lactic dehydrogenase virus
LV	leukemia virus
M	*Micrococcus* *Microsporum* *Mycobacterium* *Mycoplasma*
MDHV	Marek's disease herpesvirus
Mf	microfilaria

MLV	Moloney's leukemogenic virus mouse leukemia virus
MSV	Moloney's sarcoma virus murine sarcoma virus
MTV	mammary tumor virus
N	*Neisseria* *Nocardia*
NDV	Newcastle disease virus
O	nonmotile
O&P	ova and parasites
P	*Pasteurella* *Plasmodium* *Proteus*
Past	*Pasteurella*
PLV	panleukopenia virus
PPLO	pleuropneumonia-like organism
PS	*Pseudomonas*
PVM	pneumonia virus of mice
R	*Rickettsia* rough (colony)

**REO virus,
  reovirus**
	respiratory and enteric orphan
	  virus

RS	respiratory syncytial (virus)
RSV	Rous sarcoma virus
RV	rat virus rubella virus

S	*Salmonella*
	Schistosoma
	Spirillum
	Staphylococcus
	Streptococcus
SGV	salivary gland virus
SH virus	homologous serum-transmitted hepatitis virus
SLEV	St. Louis encephalitis virus
SLR	*Streptococcus lactis,* resistant
STAPH, Staph	*Staphylococcus*
STR, STREP, Strep, strep	*Streptococcus*
SV, SV 40	simian virus
T	*Taenia*
	Treponema
	Trichophyton
	Trypanosoma
TB, Tb	tubercle bacillus
TMV	tobacco mosaic virus
TP	*Treponema pallidum*
TV	*Trichomonas vaginalis*
V	*Vibrio*
VSV	vesicular stomatitis virus
WB	Willowbrook (virus)

Other titles of related interest from
MEDICAL ECONOMICS BOOKS

Isler's Pocket Dictionary of Diagnostic Tests, Procedures & Terms
Charlotte Isler, R.N.
ISBN 0-87489-189-2

Medical Phrase Index
Jean A. Lorenzini
ISBN 0-87489-198-1 (paper)
ISBN 0-87489-149-3 (casebound)

Simplified Medical Dictionary
Richard Franks and Harry Swartz, M.D.
ISBN 0-87489-054-3

Guide to Surgical Terminology, Third Edition
Frances Coleman
ISBN 0-87489-191-4

Medical Word Building
ISBN 0-87489-043-8

The Language of Medicine: A Guide for Stenotypists
Elsa Swanson Cooper
ISBN 0-87489-045-4

For information, write to:

Customer Service Manager
MEDICAL ECONOMICS BOOKS
680 Kinderkamack Road
Oradell, New Jersey 07649